THE ALZHEIMER'S FAMILY MANUAL

Advice for the Caregiving Journey

Lyle Weinstein

2nd edition

Copyright © 2015 Lyle Weinstein

All rights reserved

ISBN 9781511743464

BISAC: Health & Fitness/Diseases/Alzheimer's & Dementia

The Alzheimer's Family Manual

Dedication

To my father,

whose journey continues to impact me and my sisters decades after his passing.

To my mother,

whose own journey as a caregiver transformed her.

To the more than 5 million Alzheimer's patients in the United States

and the many millions elsewhere, now and in the future,

who can only benefit from the kindness of genuine caregiving.

The Alzheimer's Family Manual

The Alzheimer's Family Manual

Table of Contents

Dedication..ii
Preface vi
Introduction viii

Part I
The Alzheimer's Family Manual Audiotape Text..............1

Part II
Caregiving 47

    Caregiving as a Spiritual Discipline....................47
    Caregiving Ethics..56
    On Medical Intervention................................82
    On the Right to Die.......................................87
    Children's Issues..96

Part III
My Father 105

Part IV
Contemplating Alzheimer's..125

Afterword...145

Resources 147

The Alzheimer's Family Manual

The Alzheimer's Family Manual

Preface

My father started showing signs of Alzheimer's Disease (AD) at the age of 54. He hid them, somewhat successfully, for a few years. My mother took care of him at home for many years—until caring for him became overwhelming. He spent his last years in nursing homes with special Alzheimer's Disease units.

In 1992, during his illness, I wrote and produced an audiotape, The Alzheimer's Family Manual, to try to help other families dealing with AD. I was asked to serve on the Board of the Santa Barbara Alzheimer's Association, and in that capacity, I gave talks to caregivers and support groups for a number of years. Not long after my father passed away, I took a break from this work.

Now, more than 20 years later, those of my friends who remember that I had done this work in the past—and are dealing with Alzheimer's Disease in their own parents—have started asking me many of the same questions that came up in support groups I worked with: What should they do with the diagnosis and their loved one?

The Alzheimer's Family Manual does not purport to be a scientific study of the disease, nor is it a treatise of any kind. The intent was to create a foundation for working with loved ones in the context of this illness—both patients and caregivers, as the diagnosis and its implications are terrifying. I wanted to help enable caregivers, in particular, and their support networks to quickly get up to speed on how to protect their loved ones who have been stricken with AD, as well as each other.

Knowing that there are commonalities in patients and caregivers, and knowing that there are differences, please use whatever is in here that works for you at that moment. Set aside the rest, perhaps it will prove helpful at a different point in the journey. If you have insights that have proven helpful, please share them with other AD families directly and/or through the Alzheimer's Association.

The Alzheimer's Family Manual

Introduction

My father, Jerry Weinstein, died August 11, 1999 at the age of 70, 14 years after being diagnosed with Alzheimer's Disease. He was cared for at home by my mother for the first eight of those years. He spent the next few years in different institutions as we tried to match his changing needs to the available care facilities. His last years were spent in a facility designed primarily for mid-stage Alzheimer's patients. He died there; attended by our family, the staff of the facility, and local hospice workers.

In early 1992, my father went through a tremendously difficult period. It was a combination of the progression of his illness and reactions to different medications he was being given. I returned home after visiting with him for a week. I was both quite upset and depressed that the only relief I was able to provide for him was extremely limited and quite temporary.

I thought about what I might say if any of my friends were to call me up with news that one of their parents had been diagnosed with Alzheimer's. I sat down and began to type. I tried to put down what I would say about love, caution, fear, and the myriad of other emotions that had arisen for me and my family since my father's illness was discovered. I imagined myself, perhaps sitting in a quiet corner of a coffee shop, trying to help a friend.

I shared those writings with my siblings and a few close friends. In part, I did so because I needed to have feedback about my own anger and fear, as well as to see whether or not there was anything in the material that might benefit others dealing with the same situation. The result of that process was an audiotape program, "The Alzheimer's Family Manual."

I began to work with both the Ventura and Santa Barbara County, California Alzheimer's Associations as a volunteer, serving at times as a director for each. Because I lived three thousand miles away from my parents, I was unable to be there for them except by telephone and a few visits each year. In trying to help others who were struggling with Alzheimer's, I hoped that someone like me, living far from an ill parent, might help others as I was doing, just to keep the cosmic balance.

Each family that encounters AD accumulates their own experiences. My goal in making the audiotape was to organize and pass on my family's experience so that others might learn, more quickly than we did, what can be helpful in supporting the patient and the caregiver on a day-to-day basis, as well as what can be harmful. I wanted to help others to avoid some of the trials and errors that my family went through.

Without a doubt, the Alzheimer's Association and the support groups they organize are the most important resource for any family. In most ways, they are a far more important resource than the medical community.

However, my experience was that many people were hesitant to go to the Alzheimer's Association or to support groups, particularly when the diagnosis is first made. I am confident that this is a terrible mistake. It is when the diagnosis is first made that people need the clear information and the unconditional support provided by the local chapters of the Alzheimer's Association.

It seems that people first want to deal with the situation as privately as possible, often not even disclosing the diagnosis to other family members or close friends. They usually start reading some of the many important books filled with helpful information. Unfortunately, it is often too hard to read these books when your loved one is asking you where the keys are for the 50th time that morning. It is sometimes overwhelming reading a chapter that describes what is to come as the illness progresses. Too many people have told me that they would get to such a chapter, cry and never open that particular book again.

I thought that hearing a voice talking about how to work with the Alzheimer's patient on a "kitchen sink" level might be less intimidating than reading a book. It seemed that an audiotape might be helpful, given how much time people spend in their cars. I tried to lay out basic approaches to help all involved deal with the patient, the caregiver and each other, in a gentle, kind, and sane manner.

The tape was distributed in a limited way. It went to libraries, care facilities, and individuals, as well as different Alzheimer's Association local chapters. It was available at talks that I gave at local conferences and at support groups. After my father's death, I took time for myself and limited my formal activities with the Alzheimer's Association.

The Alzheimer's Family Manual

About fifteen years later, I started getting an increasing number of phone calls and letters from friends who were now encountering AD in their own families. I spoke to many people on the telephone and tried to give as much help as possible. I sent out the remaining copies of my tape. I began looking over my notes from talks I had given to support groups through the years. I decided to gather those notes and thoughts. This book is the result.

As I am now at an age when my father was already ill, these memories and writings take on a different quality. When I exhibit certain patterns of behavior that were always characterized as funny quirks of my father or grandfather, the need for self-examination arises. What also arises, and becomes more pressing, is the desire to pass on to others whatever I have learned that might be helpful.

This book is quite personal. It is based on the events surrounding my father's journey with Alzheimer's Disease, the impact that journey has had, then and now, on me and members of my family, as well as my experience with other patients and caregivers. I hope that whatever I have learned from these events, and from listening to others, will be of benefit.

The Alzheimer's Family Manual

Part I
The Alzheimer's Family Manual Audiotape Text

This section is the complete text of The Alzheimer's Family Manual audiotape, as it was recorded in 1992. Subheadings have been inserted for ease of reference in this written version.

Welcome. This audio program is for families. It's designed to help you when one of the members of your family is diagnosed with Alzheimer's Disease. This program will help you to recognize and respond to some of the emotional, psychological, and physical difficulties that both the patient and the primary caregiver will encounter.

My name is Lyle Weinstein. I prepared this program to share with you the experience and understanding my family has developed as a result of caring for my father, who suffers from Alzheimer's Disease. He was diagnosed with the disease about nine years ago at the age of 56, although he had begun showing symptoms a year or two earlier. Since his diagnosis, my mother, my sisters, myself and our extended families have all been coping with the effects the disease has had on my father and on all of us.

My goal is to pass on what we have learned so that you may learn quickly what can be helpful and what can be harmful in assisting the patient and those who take care of him on a day-to-day basis.

The family of each Alzheimer's patient has experiences that are similar to the ones my family has gone through. It's my hope that by listening to this, you will be able to help your loved one without having to go through an extended trial-and-error process as we did.

While it's impossible to cover every situation, the basic approaches discussed here will help you deal with the patient, the caregiver, and other family members in a beneficial and sane manner. The view presented here is that kindness and simplicity, on both emotional and practical levels, are the key ingredients for helping everyone involved.

The program will guide you in supporting the patient as well as the primary caregiver, the person who spends the most time caring for the patient. Many of the changes that will occur in the life of the patient and the life of the primary caregiver are discussed here. We will also discuss how you can help ease their difficulties and improve the quality of their lives.

Experiment with the recommendations made here, tailor them based on your own experiences. I encourage you to share your experiences, both the successes and failures, with other members of your family, with other caregivers, and with their family members through your local Alzheimer's Association support groups.

This program is not meant to replace the many helpful books that have been published by experts in this field. Those books cover certain issues, such as choosing a care facility, that cannot be condensed into this short program. Generally speaking, this program will introduce you to what lies ahead for the patient, what lies ahead for the primary caregiver, and what lies ahead for you. It is my hope that this program will help you better assist your loved one with both short-term and long-term issues. All of the suggestions made here come from examining difficult, real-life situations, to see what worked and what did not.

While everyone's circumstances are a little bit different, the basic issues remain the same. In other words, while we all have different personal situations, the general principles and approaches presented here will apply to you and your loved one. So listen to the examples, the recommendations, and the stories given here with an ear for how they relate to your situation. In them, you will find keys to help you provide caregiving and support.

For ease of reference, and because in my life it is my father who is the patient and my mother who is the primary caregiver, the patient is referred to in this program as male, the caregiver as female.

I hope this program proves helpful to you and to your loved one.

******

What Is Alzheimer's Disease?

Alzheimer's Disease is an illness which affects a person's brain and results in a progressive deterioration of that person's mental and physical abilities. People who suffer from Alzheimer's Disease lose their skills in different orders and at different rates of speed. It afflicts men and women of every race, creed, color, and national origin. It can affect people in their forties or fifties, or it may show up later in a person's life. Over time, changes in the patient will become quite noticeable as the symptoms of the disease progress from an unusual level of forgetfulness to complete confusion and disability.

The patient will show his illness primarily through his confusion. It may be expressed through anger, panic, or perhaps just physical difficulty. Sometimes he may be unable to express it at all—it's just right out there on his face.

The confusion has two principal aspects. The first is simply a very basic fear. The second is mistakes in perception. The patient's fear is based on his experience that he is losing the usual anchors people have in their lives. Since memory is what anchors us to our world and maintains our identity as a person, for an Alzheimer's patient, as he is losing his memory, he truly is losing his world.

For the patient, the loss of his ordinary connections to life may mean that he can no longer play cards, handle a checkbook, or even recognize his spouse. Sometimes he can't remember where the bathroom is. The groundlessness that an Alzheimer's patient experiences extends to every aspect of his daily life. Each moment becomes a struggle, a reminder of his increasing confusion. This is terrifying just to think about; it is more terrifying to experience.

The Alzheimer's Family Manual

Caring for an Alzheimer's Patient

Let's consider what it means to care for an Alzheimer's patient.

The realization that someone you care for has Alzheimer's Disease is a harsh one. Since presently there is no cure, the medical aspects of the illness, and the gradual deterioration of your loved one's mental and physical capacities, are realities that will not change. If and when a cure is found, it is unlikely that it will heal your loved one and bring him back as the person you knew. So the unfortunate truth is that the patient, the primary caregiver, and family members alike will all experience great difficulty dealing with the disease.

There are certain things you can do to make life simpler for everyone. There are also things that can exaggerate the difficulties and make life a continuous struggle. Again, the key elements to helping the patient are kindness and simplicity. You can help provide these from wherever you live — whether you're in the same town as the patient or 3,000 miles away.

Beyond just easing the pain you experience as a result of your loved one's illness, being part of his extended caregiver network will actually help your loved one and those who take care of him. You can help him relate to the ordinary, kitchen sink level of day-to-day life. This will help keep the illness from overwhelming everyone involved, and it will also give everyone more space and time to consider long-term approaches to the medical and emotional issues.

This is an opportunity for you to express your love and affection in ways that will genuinely repay their kindness and love for you. You actually can help them in ways that no one else can.

Family Support

The need for emotional support will arise as soon as the diagnosis is made. As a first step in establishing a plan for the patient's care, create a time and space for a family discussion to occur. Since strong emotions will arise at this first meeting, it's best not to include the patient. Be sure, however, that someone is taking care of the patient away from the meeting.

There may be completely different opinions within the family about how, or even whether to tell the patient the diagnosis, or perhaps about other steps that need to be taken. It is likely that everyone will have a strong reaction and that conflicts may arise. It will be a difficult discussion, so try to create a supportive atmosphere.

As best you can, encourage people to be gentle with each other, to say their piece, to express their concerns for the patient, their concerns for the primary caregiver, for themselves, and for others in the family. Try to express whatever fears you may have. If you do so, others will most likely feel comfortable doing the same.

Appreciate and acknowledge the confusion and pain everyone feels about the situation. This will enable you to deal with issues as simply and as straightforwardly as possible. Try to reach a consensus on the role each family member will play in caring for and supporting the patient.

After you have arrived at a consensus, meet together with the patient. Remember, simplicity is important. So one family member should present the plan you have developed together for taking care of him. Everyone's presence will help assure him that you are all there to help.

Again, you can express your basic love and affection by letting him know that you understand that he is experiencing great difficulty. Try to keep confrontations and differences of opinion among the family to a minimum, and certainly keep it away from the patient.

Reassuring Your Loved One

The patient has probably been aware that a problem exists for quite some time. Because most patients live in fear of exposing how sick they are, try to create an atmosphere of gentleness so that he has a space in which he can feel safe. Maybe he will express his fears, usually he will not. Realize that he generally cannot express them to his principal caregiver for fear that the caregiver will abandon him. Reassure him of your support, and be gentle in discussing what is happening.

There are several ways to deal with the patient's fears. First, let him know that fear is part of the illness. Because patients are frightened, they generally go through a period of denial. That's when they suspect something is wrong, but they don't know what it is. They experience difficulties with things that were never difficult before.

This might lead them to think they are going crazy. When the diagnosis is made, let the patient know that he is ill, not crazy. Even though the patient may not understand the term "Alzheimer's Disease," just knowing that his condition has a medical label can be helpful, even comforting.

Second, let the patient know that you see the fear he is experiencing and, most important, that you will stay with him, to help him through the fear of that moment. This may mean just holding his hand for a few minutes, or taking him for a walk outside for an hour. Sometimes it means being dragged up and down hallways for days on end.

Try not to panic in response to the patient's fear. If you panic, you confirm his panic. That will just provoke more panic in the patient. Don't do it.

Instead, provide reassurance that you are there, regardless of his fear, regardless of his loss of memory. Do your best to remain still and exude warmth and stability, even if you, too, feel frightened. This will help him calm down and pacify his fears. Essentially, your stability can become the stability the patient is no longer able to provide for himself.

Besides remaining calm, try to be completely present,

physically and mentally, when you're with the patient. Tell him what a good parent he is, what nice events you've shared together. Even though the patient may not remember specific events, the emotional quality of the stories and of your communication can evoke very good feelings for both of you.

So, have confidence. You can remain loving, affectionate, and strong. You can help the patient by making his world appear safe for him as he is, and safe for him as he changes.

Third, if you are far away, write letters to the patient. Send pictures of your family, of your life. The letters and pictures can be shown and read to the patient, even if he can no longer read himself. This is another way to give him more reassurance that he is not being abandoned. The letters can be saved and re-read to him by the primary caregiver whenever that type of reassurance is needed.

Mistaken Perceptions

As mentioned earlier, the patient also becomes confused and frightened because of mistakes in his perceptions. Basically, this results from that fact that he is losing the ability to coordinate information in his mind. In other words, the input from his sense perceptions happens—he can still hear, see, smell, taste, and feel—but he can't correctly put together these perceptions in his mind. For instance, he may be unable to distinguish the sound of your voice from the background sounds in the room.

Usually, mistaken perceptions are simple, like mistaking a piece of white plastic for a square of cream cheese. Sometimes the mistake in perception can occur in a potentially dangerous situation, such as while driving a car. The patient might see his child driving a car and panic, because he "knows" that the child behind the wheel is too young to drive. But what he might not put together at that moment is that his child is now 40 years old and has been driving for twenty years.

Sometimes the errors in perception become complicated because the patient mistakenly reacts with panic. This panic can get worse and worse until he has what is called a "catastrophic reaction"—a kind of panic upon panic until communication becomes impossible and there is nothing you can do to calm him down.

The key to dealing with such misperceptions is to acknowledge the patient's state of mind, not to contest his perception. Contesting his perception without giving him something else as an anchor can precipitate a catastrophic reaction. Instead, you need to provide warmth and calmness so that the patient will relax.

What you are trying to accomplish is to have him trust your perception, even if only for the moment. Try to understand what he perceives, what he's trying to communicate, and then work around it.

If you can't, just stop. Sit still and be calm.

Remember to keep it simple—stop what's going on, go for a short walk, sit with the patient for a while and hold his hands. In the absence of a medical emergency, stopping the momentum of the confusion is far more important than arguing about whose perception is right or wrong.

The caregiver has already begun to confront these problems of the patient. In fact, this is probably why they went to the doctor in the first place. In the case of my father, he had his hearing checked six or more separate times over a three-month period. He thought he was going deaf because he was no longer able to hold a conversation. Each time his hearing was tested, it checked out perfectly.

The problem was not with his ears, which in fact were picking up the sound and sending the messages to his brain. What was happening was that he was losing the minute-to-minute memory needed to hold a conversation. He just couldn't hang on and organize the messages long enough to converse. In addition, he was losing the ability to separate out the sound of a voice from the background sounds of the room he was in.

Working with the Patient's Anger

One of the most difficult aspects of the disease to deal with is the patient's anger. He may become angry when a connection he struggles for in a conversation is challenged, even in a gentle way. It is better to agree with the patient, again avoiding a catastrophic reaction. Agreement does no one any harm, even if it might qualify as a "white lie." In fact, it can be completely kind in itself, and can pacify a tense situation. Otherwise, you may end up arguing about who is right. That will just upset him more.

So trust yourself and your relationship with the patient. That will enable you to help the patient with his fears. It will enable you to avoid taking the patient's confusion personally when it comes out as anger or frustration. It's not a personal attack on you. The patient does not form the intent needed to personally attack anyone. His anger is a product of the illness and of his own confusion.

Families who care for a loved one with Alzheimer's Disease always have their share of stories. They usually revolve around the difficulties and effects of the patient's illness. The drama of the stories is not important, but the solutions they contain often show what works and what does not. They offer clues to providing active kindness. Here is an example.

My parents had a dinner party one evening. I was there along with my father's brother and his wife, as well as two old friends. My father did not say a word for virtually the entire meal. This was the time when he was beginning to have a lot of trouble following conversations. There were too many people for him at the dinner table, even though they were all familiar. The problem was exaggerated because, instead of the conversation being one on one, everyone was talking amongst each other and, as always happens in a dinner conversation, they were often speaking at the same time. It was obviously difficult for him.

The Alzheimer's Family Manual

Toward the end of dinner, someone mentioned my mother's mother, Sarah. She had died some twenty years earlier. My father sat up straight and said with a completely warm smile, "Sarah was a wonderful woman. She was always kind to me." My mother smiled and agreed. At that point my father got very upset and started yelling at her. As far as he was concerned, my mother should not be talking because she didn't even know Sarah. When she said, "But honey, Sarah was my mother," my father insisted that she was lying because she had never met Sarah. My mother then agreed with him.

Later, after the guests had left and my father went to sleep, she cried. Her tears were for many reasons—for the genuine affection my father had expressed about her mother, for his loss, and for her own loss.

From my mother's point of view, she realized that while she obviously knew her own mother, it didn't matter. My father had expressed affection at the memory of someone dear to both of them. While it was painful that he could no longer put it together that she was Sarah's daughter, it made my mother happy that my father had experienced a joyful memory of her mother. From my father's point of view, he was right. The sixty-year-old woman with gray hair across the table from him that day had most certainly never been with him and Sarah when Sarah was alive.

The anger my father expressed was not a personal attack toward my mother. What happened was that he finally felt that he could connect with the conversation. He became angry when the connection he had struggled for was challenged, even in a gentle way.

The anger he was experiencing didn't change the affection he felt for his dead mother-in-law or for his wife, but by agreeing with him, my mother avoided a catastrophic reaction. Her agreement harmed no one. Had she insisted on arguing about who was right, it would have made him even angrier. It would have stopped all communication with him and paralyzed the conversation at the table until he calmed down. He would have felt awful and more frightened about exposing himself and his illness.

As far as the other people at the table were concerned, if they had all lapsed into a heavy silence, my father again would have been confronted harshly with having made a mistake. It would have exaggerated the confusion that he already felt. If someone had leapt into the silence and started talking mindlessly to fill the space, my father would have picked up on that as another sign of his failure.

I assured the guests that everything was okay. I did that so my mother would not have to explain herself, explain the approach she had taken, or comment at all on the interchange to the other people at the table. I held my father's hand. That helped him calm down further. Then I continued the conversation in the same tone as before the explosion.

It helped my father for everyone to refrain from contesting his memory, it helped to hold his hand, and it helped to speak calmly. It helped to resume the conversation in the same tone of voice, which assured him that what had occurred was not a big deal. It helped my mother to share her pain after the event in a safe way. It's important to remember to give the caregiver the space to express her own strong and sometimes conflicting emotions.

When anger arises like that, faster than you can avoid it, it's best to just sit still and let it happen. It is never worthwhile to get caught arguing about who's right and who's wrong. Anger and frustration will arise in connection with the patient, and it will arise in connection with the caregiver. There's no question about it. Dealing constructively with it will help the patient and the caregiver. The question is how to sit still in the middle of anger and frustration.

When the patient expresses anger or confusion, you can begin by slowing down. Try to deal with it by viewing the larger situation. Ultimately, the world is not going to change if the patient confuses who you are or what your relationship is to him. It is so important to keep in mind that the patient is experiencing tremendous confusion, and that his anger arises from that confusion. His frustration is not a personal attack toward you or anyone else. Listen to him and communicate with soft words and held hands. Look directly into his eyes so that he knows you are right there with him.

When you spend any time with a patient during a catastrophic reaction, you understand what caregivers experience. Caregivers and patients go through it often.

When you're with the patient, do what you can to eliminate anything in their environment that might provoke a catastrophic reaction. Avoid bringing things to a painful point.

Of course, you should understand that there will be times when nothing works. You may not be able to pacify the situation or calm down the patient. The primary caregiver and you will just have to let the patient go through the event and have his difficulties, perhaps extreme difficulties. As this occurs, the calmer you remain, the easier it will be for the patient to calm down.

There will be times when you may be unable to remain calm yourself. This is normal, sainthood is not required.

Know that there are going to be times when you will get upset in front of the patient or with him. Be kind to yourself. Don't get angry at yourself for getting angry at the patient. Just breathe out and let go of the anger. Let go of the anger toward the patient, toward the caregiver, and toward yourself. The patient will probably forget it in a short time, so you should as well. The anger and frustration are natural reactions. It's okay to have them, it is going to happen anyway. Just don't make a big deal about it.

Staying Still

Many difficult situations can be avoided by staying still, physically and emotionally. Making a mistake for an Alzheimer's patient is not a big deal if the mistake is forgetting a name or a face. It is a big deal if the patient forgets his way home. It is a bigger deal if the patient is driving and forgets what a red light means. While each type of situation simply involves a patient making mistakes, each one results in different problems for the patient and for others, and they need to be addressed differently.

First, let's go through a situation such as a mistake of speech or a failure to recognize someone. As we said before, your reaction to this type of mistake can comfort the patient in his difficulty or it can create a further difficulty for him. If you make a face which expresses your tension, it will put more pressure on him.

There is no way around it. It is painful when your loved one looks at you and hasn't a clue who you are, or yells at you to get away. Just try to stay still in your own body, speech, and mind. Remember that it won't help the patient or you to react in kind. Ordinarily, if someone says something nasty to you, you feel hurt or angry, because you take it personally. That is not appropriate here.

The comment a patient makes is not a personal attack, it just sounds that way. What the patient is trying to express does not necessarily come out through his words. The nature of the illness limits his ability to express his confusion clearly, so it comes out in misdirected ways.

There will be times when, by accident or because you lose control, you may raise your voice to the patient, or move your body or make faces in a way that indicates irritation. It might happen with your simple desire to correct the patient or it might be the result of your frustration. An irritated, judgmental expression on your face or an angry tone of voice will accentuate the panic a patient feels. Try to slow down.

Again, don't worry about who is right or wrong. View the situation as an opportunity to communicate your love and affection. You can show the patient that it's okay that he's sick, and that your love will not disappear. You can communicate that yes, he is sick, but that's really as far as it goes. In other words, the illness can't destroy your relationship or your love.

Your concern and affection will be there whether he is a little sick, or very sick. Whether he displays his illness or tries to hide it. Your love and support, which you show by going for a walk or holding a hand, is much more important in the larger picture than whether or not he remembers a name or a word—or even you for that matter. When you treat the patient that way, it encourages his relaxation.

Try to remember what has pacified the patient in other situations and what has gotten him more upset. Remember how much a hug has meant to you when you yourself were panicked, upset, or perhaps unable to express your emotions. That's multiplied a thousandfold with the patient.

Don't be afraid to see the humor that occasionally results from the patient's confusion. Sometimes laughing will help the situation. Sometimes the patient will relax and join in. Don't feel guilty. While the humor is often very bittersweet, it's not always cruel to laugh.

The most important thing to realize and come back to is that you are a source of genuine help to the patient. You can support him in facing the effects of the illness directly. By letting him know you will not abandon him, you can immeasurably ease his difficulties.

This is, and will continue to be, an extraordinarily rough situation. There is no real time frame with Alzheimer's Disease as there is with terminal illnesses, where you usually know that it will be over in so many months or years. Patients with Alzheimer's Disease do not die from this illness, they die from other medical problems. This illness and its effects on the patient, the caregiver and the entire family, don't let up. This is a long-term situation.

Unlike the primary caregiver, you are not with the patient every hour of every day. Rouse yourself as you go to be with the patient. When you see him, bring your feelings of warmth and affection. Save your sadness for later, when you are away from him. Set up your own support network with other shoulders to cry on away from the patient's environment.

You wouldn't be listening to this program unless you cared for the patient, so always go back to that caring feeling—it is the basis of your relationship with him. Your relationship is not dependent on the status of the illness, and will not end if your parent forgets your name or no longer recognizes you. Your father will always be your father, your mother will always be your mother. Their heart always remains. The love does not stop, not yours for the patient, not his for you.

Communication

Communication with the patient is a difficult but crucial issue. As we said, most patients are afraid to expose how sick they are, or even that they are sick at all. This is particularly true at the beginning stages of the illness, but it does not stop when the illness is diagnosed. Patients continue to try to hide how sick they are. Because their own brains are functioning less smoothly, patients take their behavioral cues from the people around them. While we all take cues from another person's body language or tone of voice, for an Alzheimer's patient these cues take on greater and greater importance.

So in dealing with the patient, you need to be mindful of your body and your speech patterns. Use body language and tones of voice that communicate comfort and warmth. More and more, your most direct communication with the patient will be on this level. If nothing else is communicated, you'll let the patient know that he's in a safe place and with a safe person. This will act as an anchor for him and help him to relax.

Be mindful when speaking to the patient. Try to keep conversations one-on-one as much as possible. Remember that it isn't necessary to speak to him like a child. In fact, don't. That type of speech pattern and tone of voice will provoke anger—just speak directly, gently, and clearly.

Speak in short sentences that express one thought at a time. When you use the word "and" or the word "or" to link more than one thought, you make communication much more taxing for the patient. Ask questions that can be answered with a yes-or-no. Do not, for example, ask, "Do you want a muffin or toast?" Rather, ask one question at a time and only ask the second one if you must: "Do you want a muffin?" If the answer is no, than you could ask "Do you want toast?" It will be easier for him to answer each question separately than for him to compare muffins with toast.

Usually, we offer choices to be hospitable or gracious to others. With an Alzheimer's patient, it is often far kinder to make certain decisions for him. Rather than asking the patient, out of courtesy, if he wants butter for his bread, just give it to him if that's the way he customarily eats it. Just serve a glass of milk or a glass of juice, don't create another choice.

If you are at a restaurant and the patient either cannot or does not want to choose something for himself, just choose something for him. If he is asking you to choose for him, it is a sign that he is experiencing the choice as a test, and that he is worried about failing. So just make the decision for him and relax.

Again, the basic point here is to ease the patient's interactions with the world. Simple ideas can be very effective. For instance, encourage him to point with his finger. Pointing can be a very good method of communicating when speech is difficult. It can be helpful to the patient if you do it. It is helpful to you if the patient does it.

Giving the patient a drink with a straw is also often helpful. Because the touch of the straw is continuous and the sucking action is simple, patients often find it easier than drinking out of a glass where the angle of the glass and the level of the drink all need to be coordinated with the hands in order to make it work without spilling.

You won't always understand what the patient's confusion is. Look into his eyes. That lets him know you are there for him. It is very helpful body language. Communicate your affection and your caring. Explaining the confusion to the patient isn't relevant; communicating that making a mistake is not the end of the world is completely relevant.

Typically, if someone is telling you a story and can't find a certain word, or forgets the name of a key person in the story, you might fill in the blank and think nothing of it. When a patient forgets those things, or perhaps forgets the entire point of the story, it is a far more frightening experience both for the patient and for you. It's another reminder of the illness. It can provoke fear and panic in everyone.

Just provide the information the way you normally would, without making a big deal about it. If you cannot fill in the blank, just relax and gently go on in the conversation. Don't make a big deal about it. Don't convey the panic you might feel because you have to fill it in. Keep the situation as flat as possible by using your ordinary tone of voice and keeping your ordinary expression on your face.

Touching a patient gently can provide tremendous reassurance. Touch is a perception that is generally less subject to confusion, unlike vision or hearing. Touch is often a primary tool for communication with a patient.

For instance, you might notice that the patient will often walk a pace of two behind you, no matter how much you slow down. That is because he is unsure where he's going. So give him a reference point by holding his hand or taking him arm in arm. Touch then becomes a message of safety and reassurance. So guide him in a room with touch, rather than with your words.

Sometimes the patient will repeat the same questions endlessly. While you might get irritated, remember that the patient doesn't remember having asked it the first time, the second time, or any other time. Just answer it again, slowly. Gently change the subject. That will distract the patient but will do so in a way that reassures him of your continuing presence. That reassurance is an anchor, which is often what he is really seeking.

So remember, kindness and simplicity, gentle reassurance. These are the guideposts for helping the patient.

Supporting the Primary Caregiver

Now let's talk about the person who is most

responsible for the day-to-day care of the Alzheimer's patient: the primary caregiver. Caregivers have a different set of problems than patients. Your help in easing their difficulties will ease the difficulties of the patient. Many of the approaches we have suggested for dealing with the patient will also help the caregiver.

The primary caregiver is usually a spouse but may also be a sister, brother, son, daughter or close friend. Aside from the patient, the primary caregiver is the person who will bear the brunt of the ups and downs of the disease. She's on the front line in dealing with the changes that the patient will experience.

It's important to always remember this person. This person will be going through one of the most difficult aspect of the illness — watching their loved one, and yours, deteriorate day to day in front of her very eyes. No one is made of iron. While the type of support the caregiver needs differs from the type of support the patient needs, remember that the love and support you give to the caregiver always benefits the patient as well. Whenever you help one, you always benefit the other.

As the illness progresses, and the lives of the patient and caregiver change, your support will be needed more and more. The most important support you can provide to the caregiver is emotional, particularly when the diagnosis is first made. Your emotional support will provide strength, solace, and, whenever possible, humor. It is critical from the beginning.

Financial and practical concerns, which we will discuss later, can and should be addressed over time. Your attention to those matters can be invaluable. Dealing with those matters on their behalf enables you to support the patient and the caregiver in a different but important way.

First, we talked about the benefits of simplifying the patient's life. Simplifying life for the caregiver is equally important. Just as you need to be kind and gentle with the patient, you also need to be kind and gentle with the caregiver. For instance, a gentle touch can communicate very simply that you are there for her and that you understand her difficulties, her loneliness.

Also, consider how you can relieve, even temporarily, the stress the caregiver is experiencing. The emotional and physical health of the caregiver has a very direct effect on the health and well-being of the patient. Arrange to replace her as the primary caregiver for periods of time—a few hours, a few days, whatever you can give as often as you can give it. Make sure she gets time off from her caregiving role. Everyone's well-being depends on this kind of mutual support. Even if she insists that she is holding up fine, give her a break before she has reached the end of her rope.

Caregivers often neglect their own health as they focus on the patient. This is not good. You may need to remind her to be kind to herself, not just to the patient. Check in on her. You may need to remind her that she needs to see a doctor or to take a break. Whatever your circumstances, you have tremendous power to assist the caregiver, and you can help both of them by expressing your affection as well as helping to simplify their lives. Extend yourself as far as your personal situation will permit.

There will be times when the caregiver is at her wits end. Crises may occur over things that seem unimportant. Because you are often away from the pressures of the hour-to-hour care of the patient, you can help the caregiver to keep things in perspective. Hang in there with her when she gets upset. Again, stay still — you don't have to go up and down with the caregiver's state of mind. Just give her the opportunity to express herself; to be angry, to be upset, or to cry.

Second, schedule telephone calls to the caregiver. That way, each time she uses the phone, it isn't in the context of a crisis or panic. It can be a normal conversation. Scheduling phone calls can help eliminate a caregiver's view of herself as only a burden, which is what she may feel if phone calls only happen when she or the patient is having a particularly difficult time.

Third, write letters to the caregiver. It gives her something to show to and to talk about with the patient. Again, sending pictures of your life softens the ups and downs of the caregiver's life. It undercuts the loneliness inherent in constantly taking care of another human being.

Alzheimer's Disease creates a great deal of suffering. You cannot make everything okay, but you can help the caregiver avoid letting the disease make her own life completely claustrophobic. You can help keep her from being totally isolated.

In your letters and telephone calls, talk about the patient, talk about the difficulties the caregiver is having, but also talk about current events in your life and current events in the world. This is like opening a window in an otherwise closed room. It reminds the caregiver that life exists outside of Alzheimer's Disease.

Fourth, the caregiver may need help accepting the fact of the illness. It is not a matter of confrontation, it is a matter of clarity and kindness. You may learn from the caregiver that certain things have become burdensome. You yourself can see when the primary caregiver is being stretched beyond her limits. So take some action to lighten her load.

Some of the burdens, such as dealing with insurance companies, the checkbook, or financial planning, can be taken over completely. Some of the burdens can be shared in ways that give the primary caregiver a break—like taking care of the patient for a day, an afternoon, or even an hour.

Other ways to help are by bringing over prepared meals periodically and going food shopping with the patient and caregiver, or accompanying them to medical appointments. Deal with the outside world in as many ways as you can for the patient and caregiver. This will alleviate her sense that everything is or will become a monumental task.

Fifth, since caregivers often don't have anywhere to go or anyone with whom to speak to vent their frustration, they need to be able to talk to you about their feelings of sadness, anger, and love. This means talking someplace away from the patient. Being there for the caregiver means that when she calls or needs to talk, you are there to listen.

Again, listen to her, make sure she knows she is not abandoned and that she is not just a burden. Let her have the space to grieve, to cry for the loss of the loved one who is changing, or to be angry at whatever difficulty she encountered that day. In the same way we talked about allowing the patient the space to be sick, the caregiver also needs the space to be upset.

Family members, including the primary caregiver, usually deny the illness for some period of time. This is normal. The symptoms have shown up slowly and subtly.

Originally, the symptoms might have appeared to be the result of other factors. You might think that perhaps the patient was just depressed, or upset because he moved, sold his house, retired, or sold his business. The caregiver often participates in this denial, sometimes unknowingly and sometimes knowingly. This is because she has witnessed, initially, small behavioral, emotional, and personality changes in the patient, without having the real context to understand these changes.

In other words, the changes occurred because of an illness, not because of anything she or anyone else did or failed to do. Along with the patient, she will be afraid of what is happening and of what is going to happen in their lives. To see the illness and acknowledge it with its many ramifications is extraordinarily difficult, particularly when the symptoms of the disease are first clearly displayed. It is difficult to face the fact that your life with your loved one will never be the same.

Caregiver Stress

When the caregiver gets frustrated and angry at the patient she often ends up feeling guilty. This is true whether she expresses her anger to the patient or not. She may even feel that by having an angry thought she has been bad or disloyal.

Please assure her that a thought is nothing more than a thought, a temporary state of mind. Let her know that such thoughts and expressions of emotion are par for the course. The more she can express her frustration to you, rather than at or near the patient, the better for all concerned. Support groups are very good avenues for caregivers to express their whole mix of emotions. Encourage her attendance at a support group.

The patient's illness and confusion raises many problems for the caregiver. We just spoke about some of the ways in which you can be emotionally supportive to her.

The caregiver may exhibit signs of her temporary inability to deal with the stress she is living under. This can arise under a variety of circumstances. The pressure of taking care of the patient's needs, along with the inability to see light at the end of the tunnel, can create extreme tension and frustration. So, in addition to being emotionally supportive, there are specific things you can do in the patient and caregiver's physical environment that can be extraordinarily helpful in easing their situation.

Go through the residence with the caregiver. Notice where difficulties could arise. While you want the patient to remain as independent as possible, look at each aspect of the environment from his perspective. Physical harm—to the patient and to the caregiver—is a real issue.

The difficulties are usually just a result of the patient's confusion. For instance, stoves can be a fire hazard in the house, as well as a safety hazard to a patient. He may wander over to the stove and just fiddle with the knobs without realizing that he has just turned on a burner and is about to burn himself. If the stove is electric, perhaps a master on/off switch behind the stove, would help.

Get an electric razor instead of a blade for safety and ease of caring for the patient. Put night lights in the bathrooms and hallways. Make visual cues stronger, such as putting bright tape on a handrail and steps. At some point, it may be helpful to put a picture of a toilet on the bathroom door so as to help the patient avoid confusing the bathroom with a closet.

Make a list of these tasks but don't leave them for the caregiver to do. Just do them yourself. Everything that you do is one less task for the caregiver.

The Alzheimer's Family Manual

There are situations where the patient's confusion can result in danger to the caregiver as well as to himself. For example, Alzheimer's patients often get lost. You should get an identification bracelet for the patient. Since they often forget the meaning of traffic signals, they should not be driving. You can help the caregiver deal with the driving issue by selling one of the family cars if the patient and caregiver have two. You tell the patient that his car has broken down and had to be towed away, and therefore he can't drive it anymore. That will keep some of his anger focused away from the primary caregiver.

Going to a doctor involves being in a public place. Waiting in public places can be an exercise in fear and embarrassment for both the caregiver and the patient. The patient may have extreme difficulty waiting to see a doctor. His normal agitation will increase tremendously in a waiting room. The car ride itself may be too much for the patient, or it may be too much for the caregiver to both drive and pay adequate attention to the patient.

If a patient's confusion results in a catastrophic reaction while in a car, there is danger to the patient, the caregiver, and everyone else on the road. Try to take care of these matters when you are with the caregiver. Having an extra person along can literally be a lifesaver. It enables one person to focus completely on the patient in the car while the other drives. It enables one person to wait for the doctor to become available while the other takes the patient around the block for a walk.

Speaking to Others

From time to time, people may say insensitive things to the patient or caregiver out of their own ignorance. People who have been long-time friends may gradually become less available as a result of their own fears. This contributes to the isolation and loneliness that caregivers and patients experience.

Speak to those people directly. Explain the situation and suggest how they might help. Perhaps they could prepare a meal or go to the doctor with the patient and caregiver. Encourage the caregiver to forgive these people. Encourage the patient as well to forgive these people. Encourage the caregiver to be understanding in these situations.

Sometimes it is helpful to explain that these people may be frightened at the thought that they might be next to become sick. Old friends should be thought of kindly, even if they cannot extend themselves for the patient or caregiver now. The energy it takes to hold a grudge is much better put to use in taking care of the patient.

Helping from Afar

If you are a family member who does not live with the patient, here are some examples of things you can do even from afar that will make a difference.

The first few items have to do with taking care of financial concerns. Finances are major issues in dealing with Alzheimer's patients. Medical and non-medical care costs can be very substantial. The emotional toll which financial burdens place on the patient and caregiver's situation are enormous.

Bureaucracies are excruciating for the caregiver to deal with. The more you deal with this aspect of the outside world on their behalf, the better their days will be. Act on their behalf as an intermediary with as many bureaucracies as you can, including insurance companies, or perhaps Social Security. Get the forms each bureaucracy requires to permit you to take care of these matters. Fill out the forms so they just have to be signed by the patient or caregiver and then submit them.

Take care of filing for Medicare or Medicaid, including Social Security Disability. The more forms you fill out, the less stress on the caregiver. You may receive questions from these agencies, but remember, they actually are there to help. You will be able to arrange for additional documentation they might need and get it for the caregiver. It will be easier for you to do so than for the caregiver. That may sound strange because you could be 3,000 miles away, but the caregiver is faced with trying to get even ten minutes in private away from the patient during a single day. Not much is worse than spending that precious time waiting on hold to speak with someone.

Encourage the caregiver to go to their local Alzheimer's Association support group. Many care facilities, residential and nonresidential, sponsor such groups. It's very helpful for caregivers to know that they are not alone. Learning how other people deal with the day-to-day difficulties is helpful, and it lets the caregiver connect with a local network for help.

Many people refrain from going to support groups for various reasons. They may worry about seeing persons worse off at the moment than their loved one. They may be embarrassed. They may be unable to find someone to care for the patient while they go. Most of these problems are completely manageable.

The people organizing the support groups have experience dealing with the caregiver difficulties; they've already dealt with these problems for others and often have solutions right at hand. They will have compassion for the caregiver's situation. Encourage the caregiver to speak with their minister, priest, or rabbi. Religious groups can provide much solace as well as real practical help, including respite care or assistance with meals.

Organizing Finances

Have the Social Security checks or disability checks deposited directly into the caregiver and patient's bank account. This can be done by telephone with the Social Security Administration.

Locate the assets of the patient and the caregiver. Many people have accumulated assets over the course of their lives that they don't remember once they become ill. Many caregivers never handled the family's finances. When the patient becomes ill, he's in a very difficult situation.

If you can find records that go back before the illness struck, you will find much of the information you need. Look at old tax returns, old bank accounts, IRA statements, interest or dividend statements, or insurance policies. From a distance, you can write letters to determine whether the accounts have been closed or if they remain open, whether assets have been sold or if they still exist. You can find out if insurance policies have accumulated dividends or cash value, or even provide benefits that have not yet been applied for.

Many insurance policies generate excess dividends which are used to purchase additional life insurance. It may be that the patient now needs the income, rather than additional life insurance, at this time. Insurance policies often have cash value or can be used as collateral for loans. Many times they include waivers of premiums for cases of disability. Gather all of the information.

The patient may have securities which he has kept either at home or in a safe deposit box. Put all of them into a brokerage account. That way they won't get lost or "hidden" by the patient. In addition, in such an account all of the dividend or interest checks are collected and tracked, and can be automatically sent on to the caregiver and patient's account. This will avoid extra trips to the bank as well as the risk of losing or misplacing checks. In addition, it will make it easier to look at the overall financial situation and plan accordingly.

Get a power of attorney on behalf of the patient. There are actually two to be concerned with. One is a power of attorney to handle the assets of the patient; the second is a power of attorney to handle health care decisions on the patient's behalf when he is no longer able to speak for himself. These are effective in most states.

It's critical that the powers of attorney be secured as early as possible. It will become increasingly difficult the longer you wait. If these are not taken care of while the patient is able to express himself, the only way to accomplish the same thing is to get a conservator appointed for the patient. Getting a patient to a court hearing and having them wait in a courtroom for hours may be unmanageable as the illness progresses, so take the power of attorney route.

The asset-related power of attorney should cover all assets. Specify insurance policies, including any Veterans Administration policies, by the name of the insurance company and the policy number in the power of attorney itself.

If you don't have a family lawyer to prepare these documents, your local Alzheimer's Association has contacts in the legal community who can help with these. Also, the state and local Bar Associations often have a list of attorneys who specialize in different types of law. Look for someone who practices in the field known as "Elder law."

Put together a financial plan for the patient and the caregiver. This may be quite difficult. Many people, both caregivers and patients, do not want anyone knowing their finances. If, because of personal history or other reasons, they do not want you to help with this or even know about it, suggest that they meet with their accountant or attorney. Whenever possible, arrange meetings for them, help them to plan directly or with someone else.

Start the planning process as early as you can. It is critical to the patient's future well-being. It is also critical for the caregiver's well-being now and in the future. Make sure that the patient's attorney and accountant are aware of the patient's condition. They may be able to provide additional information and guidance.

Many people set up living trusts to hold all of their assets and income. If you can accomplish this, then the trustee, preferably someone other than the caregiver, can get all of the bills directly and pay them directly from the patient's funds. Often, a family accountant or a bank is the best trustee. They take care of the record keeping. Because they are separated from the family dynamics, they can be a helpful "outside" voice in the planning process.

Help the caregiver and patient do estate planning. Many people did their initial estate planning, if at all, long ago when tax structures were different and needs were different. Planning is important because care is very expensive. Estate taxes can be quite high and leave the surviving spouse, caregiver, or patient, as the case may be, in much worse straits than is necessary.

This is also a touchy subject in families, so it may be better to have the caregiver meet with an attorney privately, or in conjunction with their accountant.

Difficult financial issues arise for most patients and caregivers. Unfortunately, there are not many avenues to recommend. Taking care of an Alzheimer's patient is an expensive and difficult situation. Local Alzheimer's Association groups will know what service organizations exist in your area. Your local church or synagogue may be of help. Often these organizations provide respite care, perhaps free of charge — take advantage of it.

Other Issues

There are many other things you can do even if you're living quite a distance from the patient. You can stay in touch. Express your affection for the patient and the caregiver. Stay attuned to their respective states of mind. It can change day to day, month to month, and hour to hour. Acknowledge their feelings without judgment.

Be aware of physical problems the caregiver may be having. These are often the result of the tremendous stress she is under. Encourage her to take walks outside, even for a few minutes. Encourage her to sit quietly and rest for some period of time each day.

Coordinate with other members of the family or with close friends to provide the breaks a caregiver needs. Remind her that she needs a break. Caregivers often feel the need to present a strong face to the world, that they can handle all of the stress. Let her know that she can give herself a break without feeling guilty.

Visits are crucially important. Spread them out so that not too many family members come at the same time. This will limit the confusion the patient experiences when so many people are there at once. It also permits more opportunities for respite and companionship for the caregiver.

Consider a visit to where you are by the patient and the caregiver. Get as much detail as possible about what special arrangements would be helpful. Check your household. If the patient has signs in his or her house indicating the bathroom, for instance, have the same sign on your bathroom.

Keep things as simple as possible—be as normal as you can be, but perhaps a little slower, a little quieter. Remember, this is a chance to repay past kindnesses. Those don't always come around. Make sure that your children understand that their grandparent is ill, but that he still loves them. Children deal well with the patient's confusion if they are prepared in advance.

Again, make sure when you are there that the caregiver gets out on her own. When visits occur, schedule something nice for her. Get her out for tea with her friends. Send her to the market without the patient. Make sure she utilizes the respite you are offering.

Most patients have family pictures in their wallets. Some are old pictures, some may be new. Take the pictures and write in large print the name of the person in the picture, their current telephone number and their relationship to the patient. Also, cut an index card to wallet size and list all of the family members with their telephone numbers and relationship to the patient. This helps to reassure the patient, and can be a lifesaver if the patient gets lost.

Help make index cards to go on doors, drawers and cabinets. Remember that most doors look alike, most drawers look alike, and most cabinets look alike. The index cards act as memory supports which can make the day to day household life easier. Different types of cards may be appropriate at different stages of the illness.

In large block print, put on the card what item is in the drawer or cabinet or behind the door. If you can, draw a simple picture. For instance, the word glass or cup along with a picture is very helpful. The word bathroom and a picture of a toilet is very helpful. The next time you visit, bring the cards and put them up.

Schedule phone calls or write letters on a regular basis. Don't limit discussion to the patient and the illness. As we said before, sharing your life undercuts their isolation. Writing a letter to the patient can be very beneficial to you, even if he can no longer read. Writing a letter that says "I love you" to the patient often eases the loss you yourself feel.

Writing a letter to a patient or a caregiver expressing your appreciation for them - sharing fond memories — is tremendously helpful to a patient and to a caregiver. It lets them know that they are good and worthy of affection at a time when they may feel quite low due to the illness.

Remember dates that are or were important both to the caregiver and the patient. Often, it is the caregiver who will remember the dates that were important to the patient. She may become quite sad on the patient's "special" days. Send messages to the caregiver so she realizes that you have not forgotten them.

People usually remember Christmas and New Year, but the most difficult days for a caregiver are often her own birthday, the birthday of the patient, their anniversary or perhaps Valentine's Day. A phone call or visit on these days can be extremely helpful to the caregiver.

When you see the patient, start off by saying hello, and then say your name and relationship with him. This avoids tension for both of you concerning whether or not you are remembered by name. For example, "Hi Dad, it's your daughter, Linda."

Other people will need to know that the patient has Alzheimer's Disease and that the caregiver needs additional support. Tell the doctors who the patient and caregiver may see for non-Alzheimer's related illnesses. Tell other members of your extended family, your parents' minister or rabbi, and old friends as appropriate.

It can be quite difficult for the caregiver to do this. Make the call on their behalf, recommend to the person you speak with that what is needed is kindness and support — not avoidance. Pass on the recommendations contained in this program that you find helpful.

Establish your own support group. The illness will put stress on you as well as your spouse, children and other people close to you. In the same way that you should pay attention to the stress on the caregiver, ask your support group to pay attention to you.

It is important to realize that even though a task may seem small to you or to me, every task can become monumental for the patient. Every task can become monumental for the caregiver. Each time you make a telephone call, or you deal with the insurance company, that is one less thing for the caregiver to worry about.

Let the caregiver's concern be the patient. The family support group should deal with as much of the rest as possible. The more you limit the caregiver's duties to only taking care of the patient, the better off everyone will be.

Dealing with Your Own Anxiety

You will in all likelihood experience some of the same anxieties and anger that the primary caregiver experiences. Again, you can use this as an opportunity to generate compassion and kindness for the patient and caregiver. Because you experience these things, you can provide the safe outlet that the caregiver needs to express those feelings. Providing a safe outlet is critical to the well-being of the caregiver and therefore the patient.

When anger, frustration, or depression arise in your mind, deal with it directly—away from the patient and caregiver when possible. When you need to grieve, do so. Express your grief as many times as you need to. Share your grieving process within your support network. It will be beneficial to you and beneficial in all of your interactions with the patient and caregiver. And remember, your support group, as it takes on your stress, will also be affected.

Whatever you need to say to the patient, say it now. Say it as early in the process as possible. This is not the time for recriminations. This is the time to apologize for past difficulties regardless of who was to blame. This is the time to express affection.

In many ways this is the safest time to do those things. The patient has lost, or is in the process of losing, many of the habitual patterns that you may have had difficulties with. Express kindness and compassion.

Remember that when you were unable to care for yourself, as an infant for example, this person took care of you and sheltered you. Supporting the patient, the primary caregiver, and everyone in the extended family support group is based on returning this kindness.

Whether you are a lawyer, homemaker, butcher, baker or candlestick maker, you can assist in separating financial, practical, and emotional concerns, making each one less overwhelming than it will otherwise appear to either the patient or the caregiver.

The Alzheimer's Family Manual

The basic challenge is how you can help enhance the quality of life for the patient and caregiver. Advances in Alzheimer's research have yet to produce any miracle medicine to halt or reverse the effects of the disease. So it is up to all of us to help in non-medical ways. This is within our power and is far more beneficial than you might imagine.

Recommendations are easy to make. It's easy to talk about not getting frustrated or angry on the spot. It's easy to say don't feel guilty about something. To put the recommendations into practice on the spot is not always so easy. It is both the goal and the path.

In order to help the patient and the caregiver, we have to be kind. Kind to ourselves and kind to them. Kindness often means slowing down. Slow yourself down. Just because you're late for an appointment doesn't mean you should hurry the patient.

Instead, plan in advance. Give yourself more time than you think is necessary. Let the people you are going to see know that you might experience difficulties getting to the appointment on time. This is true if you are taking the patient to the doctor or to a family dinner. Just because the patient yells at you or says something apparently nasty doesn't mean that you have to yell back. Avoid being trapped by these side effects of the illness. Otherwise, you will heighten the patient's panic. Don't rush with your body, don't rush with your speech.

The Alzheimer's Family Manual

The simpler life is for the patient, the less confusion he will experience and therefore the less suffering. Simplicity will create more opportunities for sharing love and joy with the patient.

Alzheimer's Disease does not mean that your father will never smile again or that your mother will never laugh again. Alzheimer's patients and their caregivers are human beings whose lives are not over. You will learn how precious a smile truly can be. You will see opportunities for moments to genuinely share with the patient. Invite those moments. Enjoy them.

Listen to this tape periodically. Share it with other members of the family. I have included some telephone numbers on the title card so that you won't have to search for them. They include the number for the National Alzheimer's Association [800-272-3900].

If you have suggestions to make this program better or other issues which you feel should be addressed in future editions, please let us know. Thank you for listening. I hope this program will prove helpful to you and to your loved one.

The Alzheimer's Family Manual

Part II
Caregiving

Caregiving as a Spiritual Discipline

This discussion is directed to the process of caregiving as a spiritual discipline. It is not oriented to any specific illness. Instead, it focuses on the development of compassion. Genuine spiritual discipline manifests as immovable kindness and unshakable compassion, qualities which are at the heart of spirituality.

Although kindness and compassion are easy to talk about, they are not so easy to embody. A good caregiver needs to have those qualities, but how do we develop them? It is clear that those qualities can spontaneously arise in any caregiving situation on a momentary basis. However, without cultivation, they are not easy to maintain in a stable ongoing fashion.

The fact is that caregiving itself is a direct path to cultivating compassion. One generally starts out as a caregiver for quite good reasons. One can become a caregiver with some kind of altruistic intention and one can become a caregiver as a result of feelings of guilt, although it is generally a mix of the two. We find, whether it is for love or money, that the practice of caregiving is stronger than we think. By its nature, caregiving both points to and expresses spiritual discipline: its result is compassion and its manifestation is kindness.

For all caregivers of loved ones, and in all facets of

caregiving, there is a common thread of understanding — we have all been sick in the past and we will all die in the future. Our personal fears of sickness and death become quite exposed in the caregiving process. Because we cannot hide from our caregiving duties, because we will get up the next day and continue to care for our loved one, that very fear can be transformed into the path. It is a path that uncovers the deepest connection between our own heart and the heart of the person we care for.

It is easy to connect with a sick or dying person. We can see her journey right on her face. We can feel it in his body. We can hear it in their voices. It is in no way hidden. It is quite clear. There is no PhD required. We always have a choice of turning away in fear or extending out in empathy.

We usually sympathize with someone from a distance. We usually see ourselves as being in a different situation from the one who is ill. However, by acknowledging the experience of our own fear and revulsion at the prospect of sickness and death happening to us, we can do more than just sympathize. We can allow ourselves to touch and be touched.

Human bodies are so fragile, and there are so many ways to die. We are all subject to sickness, a sudden heart attack or an accident. No one knows when death will come. By acknowledging the truth of our own mortality, we can connect with the fear in our loved ones. Then we can truly be present for them, on the spot. That is genuine support, genuine kindness.

Practicing caregiving as a spiritual discipline means doing that very hard work of boycotting one's own hopes and fears. The result is a sense of honesty about sickness and death. While the goal of benefiting someone who is ill is in itself laudable, there are unanticipated benefits of truly caring for another person. These side effects can profoundly change the caregiver.

The power and benefit of caregiving to the caregiver is clearly seen when you encounter ordinary people who have been thrust by love, friendship and affection into being a caregiver. They are forced to examine their own lives, their own fears. Looking at the mortality and frailty of the loved one forces the caregiver to confront all of the emotions surrounding their own relationship with sickness and death, to their loved one, and to everyone else in the constellation of their loved one's life.

Beyond that moment, in the next moment, the next day, the next week, the next month and often for many years, they open further to the suffering and pain of their loved one. Still, in that next moment they speak softly to their loved one. They hold their hand, brush their hair, or gently feed them dinner.

This is true discipline. In its own special way, it is the joy of discipline. It is the genuine renunciation of one's own petty desires in that moment when you have to shave your father's face, or dress your mother, or clean up after a toileting accident.

As a spiritual path, it is not restricted to the mystically initiated or the great scholars. Untrained, non-professional people are fully engaged as caregivers every day. And every day, they have the profound experience of genuinely touching another human being's life, with no demand for feedback. That simple direct contact is reward in and of itself.

We often experience the process of another person's illness from the point of view of how it impacts us. In other words, while we think, "how awful, my parent is dying," our next thought might be about ourselves. We might think, "Now I am going to be all alone in the world." We cling to this idea that we are remaining and they are leaving. Our experience of their illness isn't very direct because it remains based on our reference point of self-interest, on how their illness affects us.

Generally speaking, everyone is guided to some extent by self-interest. However, sometimes our self-interest is overwhelmed by the suffering a loved one. Sometimes it is overwhelmed by the impending loss, the impending separation we see on the horizon. In either case, at that point we are transformed.

For the first time, we begin to put the well-being of another ahead of our own. We swallow our pride of social position and clean up bodily waste lovingly. We dress and undress our loved one, brush their teeth, and, most importantly, consider what needs to be done for them the next moment, the next hour, the next day. Usually, that is as far into the future as caregivers can realistically plan.

Individuals who have never put anyone's interest ahead of their own may suddenly experience what it means to do that. Individuals who have dealt with others in a generally compassionate manner will find their skills enhanced. We may find that our compassion is conceptual whereas the smell of a dying person's body is not. Again, a transformative experience.

As fears arise and increase for the patient, this can often exaggerate one's own fears and panic. When things become difficult for the patient and/or the caregiver, thoughts such as "maybe it would better if one or both of us were dead" might arise. When thoughts like that do arise, they are usually followed by an internal judgment of guilt. Let the thoughts of anger, sadness, and guilt, all of them, simply be. If you don't feed those thoughts, they will go the same way they came—quickly and without a trace. Simply continue to take care of that next moment with the patient.

At the beginning of the AD journey, the afflicted one may be stronger than we are. If he or she approaches illness and imminent death as a process which is part of life, this cuts off the hope and fear of survival. This can support the caregiver's own self-confidence and strength. And you can do the same for them when the time comes.

This is a great lesson to witness up close. Without holding to a cushioning philosophy, understand that the illness and imminent death is a process that is part of life. You know this to be true because you see it in the course of your caregiving relationship. Simply remember that everyone in the past who was born has either already died or will die sometime in the not so distant future.

Conceptually, it is clear that death and illness will certainly strike each of us. We hope that it won't be for quite some time, but we fear that it will be before we are ready. That is not a particularly helpful approach—particularly as being "ready" is usually quite a vague notion.

Because no one truly knows the time of death, acknowledge that and begin cutting off the attachment to notions of hope and fear. Making yourself ready in that way will support and encourage the self-confidence of the patient, who in many ways is resting in your reference points.

Similarly, when the patient's fears arise, just let them arise. When patients experience and begin to express their panic, they key off of your reaction. Instead of joining in the panic, create an open and warm psychological space by word, action or simple body language. By doing so, and not panicking yourself, you can allow their panic to happen safely and without judgment.

Do your best to simply project immovable kindness, the warmth that will not run and hide in the face of chaos. It is the warmth that refrains from easy platitudes but instead provides a genuine container for the process they are going through, without praise or blame.

That container of warm immovable kindness will allow their panic to dissipate. Communicate with soft body language that you are participating in the process with them without succumbing to panic. If you panic as well, then it's like adding gasoline to a blazing fire. Don't do that. If you allow the fuel of that moment's panic to be exhausted, things will settle down.

In that same way, your "bad" or "guilty" thoughts should not be suppressed, but nor should they be a focal point for self-criticism. That is not the point. Do not forget to be kind to yourself as well. Experience such thoughts simply and directly in that same space of kindness you try to provide for your loved one, again without praise or blame.

It is helpful to understand that the experience of getting caught in those cycles of thoughts is close to the experience of your loved one. Recognize those thoughts as your hopes and fears, and let them dissipate in the same way. They arose in a moment, and they will be gone in a moment.

They might seem to exist longer than just a moment, but that will only happen if we cultivate and dwell on them. Go back to the present, whether it is preparing the next meal, going for a walk, or simply breathing. The thoughts will leave unbidden, just as they came.

Caregiving, from beginning to end, encourages an openness to experience directly the attachment to your loved one. Your attachment may appear in the holding on to hope that the patient will recover or go easily, and fear that they will pass away in great difficulty. From the point of view of the patient, see how they experience their attachment to things, recollections, and their body.

Visits with family can be wrenching for both the patient and family member(s) as a result of attachments to unfinished business as well as attachments of affection. Taking any side, trying to force resolution of issues of hope or fear will exaggerate the attachments. Don't take sides. The only side which exists is this very moment of kindness.

As life becomes undeniably more tenuous, there is no time like the present. Being present in this context means not moving when the patient's mind moves. Be with them without being trapped by them. This gives a reference point for them to return to. If they express anger, meet it softly. If they express panic, project stability. If they express desire, meet it gently. If they express love, honor it fully without grasping.

The point is to provide support in the present moment as that is truly the only moment you have. In other words, nothing can save you from the present moment, so relax any sense of struggle. In that moment, you can be true to yourself.

From the point of view of the caregiver, this requires both discipline and exertion. Hope and fear continually arise in the caregiving situation. The future, or the lack of a future, can easily become monumental obstacles for all participants in the process. Boycotting those kinds of obstacles opens up the environment for genuine communication with and without words.

The process of grieving actually starts when the diagnosis is first made. It intensifies as the illness becomes less and less hidden. It can feel overwhelming when the patient is clearly slipping away beyond any imagined hope of recovery. Nevertheless, it is critically important for the patient to have the psychological space to experience their dying process without rubbing up against the caregiver's mental tides. They will need all of their strength and waning energy to connect directly to the journey of their illness and death.

Part of the spiritual discipline of caregiving is creating open and supportive space for the patient. The boundaries of the patient's world, which become more and more intimate on both the physical and psychological level, deserve complete respect. This requires the caregiver to work with their own emotions, however conflicting, intense and swirling, separate from the patient's space.

When you are the caregiver, bringing your issues into the patient's presence drains their strength and energy. Remember that sainthood is not a prerequisite for being a caregiver. Besides, even saints experience dark nights, trials and fear. So, don't ignore the important work of caring for your own needs. Make sure you have your own support network of friends around whom you can allow upheavals to arise. Do not forget that there are others treading the same path as you, quite happy to share and support your journey.

Caregiver Ethics

This section is drawn from a series of talks that were given to caregivers first dealing with the diagnosis in their families.

There are very few "bright line" tests concerning caregiving ethics, except for protecting the patient, as best as one can, physically, emotionally and financially. There are no single answers that work for everyone. These issues and their resolutions are quite personal.

While I do not have the answers for even one other person, I do know that it is critical to look at the questions and explore how one's own feelings get provoked. It is important to encourage family members and others involved in the caregiving network to do the same. Look at the questions and feelings now, rather than in the middle of a crisis. In that way, you can sort out and clarify your own confusion—usually a mix of fear with conflicting emotions—at a calm and quiet time. This will help you to more clearly see and deal with crises when they do arise.

In caring for an AD patient, there are several choices that need to be addressed very early on. The decisions made, and the considerations that go into making them or leaving them unmade, can have profound impacts later on.

The basic view should always be grounded in simplicity and kindness. This translates into taking actions that eliminate as much chaos as possible for your loved one afflicted with AD.

The specific issues addressed here are:

1) The Diagnosis
2) Competence
3) Making Decisions
4) Institutionalization
5) Abuse
6) Unrelated Illnesses
7) Family Conflict

Diagnosis. Having trouble with memory does not necessarily mean a person has AD. Dementia-like symptoms can appear due to depression, drug interactions, thyroid problems, excess use of alcohol or a host of other causes. Symptoms based on those kinds of cases can be treated and reversed. The AD diagnosis is made by a doctor and until that diagnosis is made, the suspicions of AD remain mere suspicions. However, the moment the diagnosis is made, the amorphous fear becomes concrete.

Diagnosis of AD means that other treatable conditions have been ruled out. So, make sure that the diagnosis has been confirmed by a competent physician, one who specializes in AD, and after the necessary tests have been performed.

When taking your loved one for an evaluation, don't go alone. If the diagnosis is confirmed as AD, you may not be in any condition to drive. Often, the diagnosis is given to the caregiver rather than the patient. The idea, at least as presented to my family, is that the patient won't really understand it anyway.

While that is true later on, I strongly disagree with that approach. In my father's case, having a name for his illness made him feel safer in that it meant he didn't have to hide so much anymore. It also meant that because the doctor knew what was wrong, he wasn't simply going crazy. He didn't conceive of what would happen over the next fourteen years, but then no one in our family could.

The doctor told us that he wouldn't live more than four or five years, and that he wouldn't suffer. The doctor was wrong on both counts. There was no communication from the doctor or his staff about what really was going to happen as a result of his illness. Their only advice was, in effect, to grit your teeth and go through it.

Once the diagnosis is made, the first issue is what to say. The second issue is how to say it. My father wanted to talk to me after the diagnosis. I took him for a walk so that he could have the privacy he seemed to want. He looked at me and said, "I'm very sick, aren't I?" I answered directly and immediately, "Yes." "I'm not going to get better, am I?" "No, you aren't." He understood this simple and accurate explanation. It was irrelevant that the term Alzheimer's Disease had no meaning for him other than that there was an explanation for what was happening to him.

He asked what would happen. I gently told him that he would forget more and more things. I told him that he would likely forget my name and the names of my sisters. I also looked him straight in the eye and told him that we would be with him and take care of him whether he remembered who we were or not. I told him that we all loved him and that would be the case regardless of whether or not he recalled our names.

These things that I said were all true, and proved to be true throughout his illness. The point of the story is that by me remaining calm, soft, and honest, he felt comforted and safe. It is an extremely important lesson to understand: You may be able to provide that sense of safety. Even though it may only be for a few moments at a time, it is extremely valuable to both of you.

In telling your loved one the truth, understand that you will be their reference point. However much you were a reference point in the past, you become an even more crucial anchor as they lose the ability to maintain independent reference points of their own.

This means that maintaining your emotional stability in their presence will be extremely beneficial, but that displaying your emotional panic will be equally unhelpful. Panic all you want, grieve all you want, scream if that helps, but do it <u>away</u> from your loved one. Do it at the support groups, do it with your extended caring network, do it when you are in whatever spiritual container you may enter.

Knowing that a problem exists, and being able to discuss it, are very different things for a caregiver. Usually, the initial signs of AD are very subtle. The patient is able to hide them from view for quite some time. For their spouse or other primary partner who spends time day in and day out with the patient, it is when the initial symptoms are no longer quite so hidden that the fear of the diagnosis can be overwhelming.

Just as the patient hides his illness, caregivers often feel that they need to protect the patient by similarly hiding the diagnosis. This mistaken view must be overcome. There is nothing to be embarrassed about. Simply taking care of things as they arise is the best antidote. There is no benefit in hiding.

In telling others, first remember to be kind to yourself. Take time to process the ramifications of the diagnosis, just not in front of your loved one. Similarly, prepare family and friends for what they may encounter before they visit. You can also ask close family/friends to help prepare others for you.

Encourage everyone to leave their personal pain at the door for the benefit of the patient. Suggest how they can ease the situation by avoiding anything that smacks of a test to the patient. So, remind them to introduce themselves rather than opening with, "Do you remember who I am?"

Competence. From the point of view of the law, definitions of mental competence vary from state to state, and from country to country. Definitions also vary as to the circumstances under consideration. Competence in criminal matters may differ from competence in civil matters such as contracts, wills, and powers of attorney. Competence for purposes of probate, powers of attorney and the like, is analyzed based on a series of factors. Competence is presumed but that presumption is rebuttable.

Taken alone, the AD diagnosis does not necessarily mean that someone is incompetent for these purposes.[1] One must take into account a person's orientation to time, place, person, and situation, as well as their ability to concentrate and process information. Short-term and long-term memory, including immediate recall, is a relevant concern, as is recognition of familiar objects and persons. In addition, one must analyze the ability to reason using abstract concepts.

Legal definitions of competency are critical for documents that give authority for actions to be taken on behalf of someone when they cannot communicate their wishes on their own, or when their wishes are clouded by their illness. These documents are extraordinarily helpful, but there can be periods of time when competency is not so clear-cut. The longer you wait to deal with these issues, the more the risk increases that the progression of AD will render the patient incompetent.

When looking at the issue of competency, remember how important environmental cues can be to someone with AD. There are many people in good health that panic walking into a lawyer's office. Consider how much more frightening it might be for someone with AD.

Taking the patient to an unfamiliar and frightening lawyer's office may well determine whether the documents can be legally executed, as the determination of competency is made at the moment of signing the papers. It may be less

---

[1] California Probate Code Sections 810-813

stressful to have the attorney come to the patient's home or some other familiar environment in order to discuss and execute such documents.

Once AD starts to display its more profound effects, one needs to consider whose wishes are really being looked at. For example, my father was always explicit about his wish to have no extraordinary actions taken to prolong his life. He said this many times, but it was always about "pulling the plug" should he be on life support. He always emphasized that his fear of living as a vegetable or semi-vegetable far exceeded his fear of death. These conversations took place before AD was a commonly known illness. The instruction about not taking actions to prolong his life were never in the context of a long-term illness that would rob him of his mental capacity in a slow but inexorable way.

Following his AD diagnosis, and for at least two years after, he hid the growing symptoms. During this period, his historical reference points about death began to dissolve. Fear of people close to him taking his possessions and his money arose for the first time. Fear of dying took on monumental qualities that never existed for him before.

One can reasonably ask which view of my father should control at that point in time—the view of the pre-AD person I had known all my life, or the one now fully in the grip of the disease? These were extremely different views.

This is not a philosophical question based on hypotheticals. It was a very real and intensely personal situation with strong pulls in many directions. For a family, this is often exacerbated by the fact that not everyone will necessarily agree with each other.

These changes can bring about extremely painful situations. Your loved one will be asked by an attorney, doctor, care facility staff, or family member about their wishes concerning the terms of a Durable Power of Attorney for Health Care, a will, or a financial power of attorney. When they look to you, do you honor the patient's historical view or his current view? Do you encourage what you think is appropriate now, or what you think will be appropriate when competence is clearly no longer even in question? Do you refrain from giving your loved one any cues at all on these questions, even though you know this will generate even more fear for him? The permutations appear endless and without a comfortable resolution—whatever decision is made.

Practically speaking, by maintaining a soft emotional atmosphere, one can include options that are appropriate now as well as those that will work later. You can set the stage for either a gentle transition of control, or you can create obstacles and battles. Remember, executing the documents requires competence at the time they are signed. Only with that then-current competence can the documents be enforced later.

If people in the caregiving circle cannot agree, start with whatever points are in agreement and try to build bridges from there. There may come a point where a decision has to be made that cannot be made unanimously. This often happens when the decision may be extremely painful or abhorrent to someone in the circle.

Again, there are no hard and fast rules. However, deference needs to be given to the wishes of the primary caregiver, the one who is on call morning, noon, and night. That person is the one on whom the greatest burdens will lie. With that deference, and using a gentle tone, everyone needs to be supportive to the extent they are capable.

For family members living far away, or who are unable to contribute much to the daily care of the patient, there can be a tendency to feeling guilty. In compensation, they can be more officious and obsessed, insisting that everything has to be done for the patient to an unreasonable degree, or in some other way trying to micromanage the care and the primary caregiver from a distance. Understanding that this is an expression of both love for the patient and an overcompensation to assuage guilt, one can avoid potential antagonism that will in no way benefit your loved one.

Making Decisions. Making a decision for an adult, especially one who is your parent or spouse, is not an easy task. Outside of one's children, when they are very young and can still be told what to do, or for someone in military service, we generally don't make all that many decisions that truly will control someone else's life or death. Decisions for AD patients must take into account the impact on the patient and the primary caregiver.

Is the decision based on a recollection of what your loved one would have wanted when they were well? What they want now? What you think would be best for them? Or maybe what you think will enable you to continue to care for them? While there are many questions, again there are no hard and fast answers. The purpose of raising questions here is to encourage everyone's ongoing dialogue, both with each other and internally within oneself.

There are several contemplations recommended in Part IV of this book that may enable you to feel the texture of your mind as it would react to various options that might be chosen for you. With that, you can gain insight into how your loved one might react, both positively and negatively, as well as how you might best proceed.

Kindness and simplicity, as always, are the guideposts here. With those in mind, consider some of the critical issues that arise for almost every AD patient and their family. How and when do you take away someone's license to drive? After an accident or simply after a near miss? Immediately after the diagnosis, or when you think it might be starting to be noticeably dangerous?

There is the delicate balance between taking away a prime indicator of independence, such as a driver's license, when a loved one may be grasping tenaciously at it, and protecting them from themselves. This situation is complicated further when the primary caregiver is the one holding on to that indicator of independence.

My father didn't want to drive much after his diagnosis. However, he did not want to give up his driver's license. My mother felt that to simply take it away would have been a brutal show of force exposing how ill he was.

When my mother told me that he had recently stopped in an intersection, uncertain if he was supposed to go straight, left or right, I removed the distributor cap from his car. I simply told him that the car wasn't working and that we would fix it soon. He went out to look at the car for about three days in a row, tried the key a few times but nothing happened. As my mother always drove her own car, there was not a huge problem. After a few weeks, he stopped asking about it. Then, we got rid of the car altogether.

To time exactly when it is "too" dangerous for them to drive is impossible. There are risks to the patient, whoever is in the car with them, whoever is sharing the roads, and even people simply walking on the street.

My grandfather, who exhibited many symptoms of AD but was never diagnosed, drove himself and my grandmother until we realized that he was a danger on the road to himself and others. This was true even though he was only driving a few blocks back and forth to the supermarket at that point. It took a while to understand the danger because either my father or I drove when we were with him.

Nevertheless, one day I was in the passenger seat when he failed to notice someone jay-walking across the street. When I pointed out the man and suggested that my grandfather slow down, his response was to say that the man wasn't supposed to be crossing there anyway and he hit the gas. We took away his car immediately. After a slight argument, he relaxed and admitted that he felt frightened driving. The only reason he kept driving was that my grandmother insisted.

These same concerns arise with many other ordinary day-to-day activities. The kitchen is a dangerous place for an AD patient, just as it is for a child, and simply crossing streets becomes a concern. For your loved one, get an identifying bracelet with home address, telephone number and vital information, including the AD diagnosis.

Protection is critical not just of the patient but also of the caregiver and innocent bystanders. All of these come up in the driving context, and often in the cooking context.

Diverting your loved one's attention is often the simplest and safest route to take. Removing the distributor cap is an example of that. When my father asked if we needed to have someone fix the car, of course I said yes, we did, and I would invite him to go for a walk. That satisfied him. At that stage of the disease, he would not remember having had the conversation with me five minutes later.

Remembering requires the ability to conceptualize, an ability that is eaten away by the illness. One must take a direct approach to the real concern — establishing a sense of safety for your loved one. If they feel safe, diversion is easy. If they don't feel safe, it is much more difficult.

Physical contact is usually very persuasive. If they want to drive somewhere, it is pretty simple to hold their hand and ask them to take you for a walk, or ask them to listen to some favorite music. Also, don't say "Wouldn't you rather..." or "Instead of going for a drive..." — phrase it as a direct statement — "Let's go for a walk together." It is much easier for an AD patient to understand.

The same question of balancing concerns about safety with concerns about unduly impinging on the patient's control over his life arises with medication. Often, a drug will mimic the effect of the illness while calming some of the difficult externalized behaviors. The side effects of many AD prescribed medicines include an inability to concentrate, trouble with speaking, loss of coordination and so on. All of these can also be symptoms of AD. As such, the medications will affect the ability to gauge how severe the impact of the illness is on the patient at any point in time.

Such medicines may be necessary to preserve the sanity of the caregiver. Sometimes they are necessary to help the patient get through the day. Sometimes it is not clear which reason predominates, or which reason should predominate. What should always remain clear is that treating external behavior is not a substitute for genuine caring affection.

While physicians do not serve as your personal support network, they are there to help. They are an adjunct expert for you as a caregiver and for the caregiving support circle around you. Please ask, firmly and repeatedly if necessary, the names, dosages, intended effects and possible side effects of any prescription medication. This will help you support your loved one.

I must insert here another plug for the Alzheimer's Association support groups. These support groups are often the only context in which you will be alerted to certain information. Often, it is only through communicating with those going through the same journey that one can actually discuss the issues one is facing.

For instance, sexual issues are often difficult to discuss. This is true for many people regardless of sickness or health. What you may not know is that some of the drugs prescribed for AD patients have side effects on their sexuality. This is not something that one would necessarily think about when administering medication to your loved one, but it may end up being extremely difficult for you to manage.

Other drugs have side effects which mimic the symptoms of AD, as discussed earlier. Understand that they are often prescribed for patient management, rather than symptomatic relief. You may indeed need them for managing your loved one, but it's also possible that you may not.

When my father was having difficulties that I suspected were drug related, I took a dose of one of his prescriptions. It was an anti-psychotic drug sometimes prescribed for AD patients, despite the fact that AD is not a psychosis.[2]

I was told by my doctor that it would not affect me in the same way as it affected my father because I did not have AD. Nevertheless, after being warned not to drive or go anywhere outside my house (and being given his home number to call if there was any emergency), I took it. I went through 20 to 30 minute cycles of complete exhaustion followed by passing out for that same amount of time and then awakening with such a jarring sensitivity to stimuli that I wanted to absolutely not move.

That experience made it completely clear why this drug had been prescribed to my father and others in his AD facility. It had nothing to do with treating my father's AD. It had everything to do with managing him as a patient. So long as he was paralyzed by medically induced exhaustion and extreme sensitivity to stimuli of any kind, he would not wander or cause any trouble. The drug was removed from his prescription list at my insistence. Perhaps there is a reason for prescribing this for AD patients that has a real benefit for them. I personally doubt it.[3]

Pharmacology is not the only physician related concern. Some doctors do not have experience with AD patients. Again, as the caregiver, you are the patient's last

---

[2] I do not recommend this to anyone. There are dangers in taking any medication, particularly one that is not prescribed for you. Further, different people react to the same medication in very different ways, sometimes because one person does not have the targeted illness, sometimes because the individuals have different metabolisms.

[3] The drug in question now carries a warning of the risks of giving this to a dementia patient but does not prohibit it.

line of defense.

Many years after my father had lost the ability to speak, much less comprehend speech, he was hospitalized. A doctor came in to tell him that they were going to perform a spinal tap to make sure that there was no infection in his spinal fluid. He cautioned my father that when he woke up from the procedure, he should not move at all for two hours in order to avoid complications.

Fortunately, my mother was in the room. She told the doctor that he needed to speak to her about the procedure. He refused and simply repeated everything to my father. My mother pointed out that my father had AD, that it was noted on his hospital chart, and that he didn't understand a word the doctor was saying to him.

Further, she pointed out that he couldn't remember what happened moments ago and would certainly be incapable of remembering not to move post-spinal tap. The doctor became angry and left. The procedure was never done.

Not all doctors are like this. In general, doctors who work with AD patients understand the illness. However, as the caregiver, one needs to ensure that the procedures the doctor wishes to use, while appropriate for non-AD patients, are appropriate in the AD context.

Institutionalization. The issue of institutionalization arises both in the mind of the caregiver as well as in the mind of the patient. There are at least two separate aspects to take into consideration. One is the question of the quality of care in a facility, the other is the question of abandonment.

The same cautionary remarks concerning doctors extends to care facilities. The people who spend the most time actually caring for the patients are neither doctors nor nurses. It is usually the lowest paid staff that truly attend the patients.

See how these staff members are with the residents. If they speak in gentle voices, if they hold patients' hands and gently lead them, if they look at them softly and with kindness, it is likely a good place. If they do not look at the patients with softness in their eyes or give them verbal instructions without gentle guidance by touch, avoid such a place.

Don't be deceived by expensive facilities. They are often built from a marketing point of view, to convey to the families that the facility is a nice place that you won't feel uncomfortable visiting. However, your loved one won't notice it as the disease progresses. Look at the staff attendants. They are the key indicator.

If staff speaks loudly or harshly to residents, if they are generally gossiping with each other and ignoring the residents, except when one has an accident or freaks out, avoid the facility. Avoid it if it smells bad. Facilities smell bad because patients are not cleaned up right away when they have accidents.

Fears of abandonment may or may not be real. In the minds of some family members, institutionalization is equivalent to abandonment, and for some individuals, that may be true. It will depend on when and how it occurs, but primarily it depends on what happens afterwards.

Institutionalization does not by itself mean the end of a relationship. Rather, it means the relationship has changed. Usually it is the acknowledgment of a change that has already occurred. As a caregiver, look clearly at your own confusion, at your own heart. That is where your answer will lie.

A neighbor had watched my parents' difficulties grow as my father's illness progressed. She saw the difficulties he experienced while still living at home, and saw the difficulties my mother experienced when my father was later residing in a care facility. Her own husband of forty plus years was diagnosed with AD about ten years after my father, and within a month she took him to the same care facility. She dropped him off and never went back to see him. He died six months later.

Some people were horrified by this, and some still are when they hear the story. But before demonizing this woman, consider that my father continued to suffer for another four years, a total of fourteen years post-diagnosis. This other gentlemen died about six months after he was diagnosed.

This neighbor had six months of suffering with AD without his wife visiting him. My father had fourteen years with my mother's ongoing care and visits. I don't believe that anyone can say with certainty which decision resulted in less suffering for the AD patient.

Perhaps my father lived so long because my mother didn't tell him it was okay to leave. In visiting him four to seven times each week, she was communicating that she couldn't let go. At the end of every visit, she told him when she would be back. Perhaps he felt that if she couldn't let go, then he shouldn't.

A few years after this other gentleman died, my mother took my advice and ended each visit with my father by telling him she loved him and that it was okay to leave. He died a few months after that.

I cannot imagine that it was easy for the neighbor's wife to take the approach she did. One must consider the possibility that it was kinder of that neighbor's wife to have given him an extremely firm message that it was time to go. Perhaps simply telling him that it was okay to go would have been sufficient. However, I think she was quite frightened by my mother's extended journey and may have felt that any less brutal option would be too risky, even though it was likely quite brutal to herself as well.

Abuse. The issue of abuse can also be complicated. There are several contexts of potential abuse to be aware of. Abuse can occur both by the caregiver and to the caregiver. How long ought you to let your mother be hit or pinched, or for your father to scream and curse at your mother? What should be done when you are the victim of the abuse? What should be done when out of your frustration, you become the abuser?

If you notice the primary caregiver or the patient with black and blue marks, or about to explode with anger, physical intervention is critical. Closing one's eyes and hoping for the best will only lead to permitting further abuse. Make sure at the very beginning that everyone in the caregiving circle is aware of the possibility of abuse in both directions. That way, one can hopefully intervene as things become difficult—before it gets to the level of abuse.

If you are the primary caregiver, check in with support groups. If you are a concerned family member, help get the caregiver into a support group, perhaps by inviting them to a meeting that you could attend together. There are many methods for intervention, check with your local Alzheimer's Association for more information.

All caregivers lose their tempers at times. All AD patients have "catastrophic reactions" at times. There is a great deal of stress on all involved. Knowing this, it is important to take steps to train in de-escalating stressful situations. This is needed to avoid stress turning into abuse.

Don't believe that it is a flaw to seek help and support. Help exists and can lend you strength when you need it. Your strengths and insights can also help others. Experience is the best teacher and resource. Seek it out from others, and share your own.

Abuse can happen in other contexts as well. Finances are a ripe area for abuse. The possibility of financial abuse by a caregiver or financial manager is not to be taken lightly.

People with limited economic resources are often eligible for ongoing insurance payments, government support and so on. Such people, as well as people with substantial resources, can become targets for unscrupulous caregivers.

Heirs often get into disputes about whether money should be expended on a patient, or be preserved for themselves. There are also unrelated individuals who simply look to prey on the elderly and infirm when they cannot defend themselves.

In situations where this kind of abuse is suspected, courts and public advocates can be brought in. While the decisions made by such an outside process may not be palatable to the participants, they are made without any regard for competing self-interests. The associated accounting and reporting obligations that can become expensive are not an unreasonable price to pay for eliminating financial abuse in a caregiving situation. Sometimes the mere threat of court appointed trustees can quell intra-family financial wrangling.

Unrelated Illnesses. Decisions need to be made regarding treatment for non-AD illnesses. Some of the situations are fairly straightforward. A broken leg is different than systemic cancer. Certainly, to ease the suffering of broken bones is not an ethical problem.

However, there are three other broad categories that one needs to consider in advance so as to establish action plans should the circumstances arise: long-term systemic illnesses such as cancer, short term illnesses that left untreated can be fatal, and immediate crises such as strokes.

Discuss and decide the course of action before the event, not during it. During the event, support the patient and primary caregiver through the entire process, whatever decisions have been made. Making decisions in the middle of a medical crisis engenders guilt, which can result from either letting someone go <u>or</u> from keeping them alive.

While making decisions before a crisis will not avert all feelings of guilt or second thoughts about the actions taken, there is a sense of having balanced the relative qualities of the potential choices. While there may never be a "good" choice that everyone agrees incontrovertibly avoids the most suffering, one can have confidence that the decision that was made was fully considered.

None of us can see the future all that clearly, and weighing relative suffering is never an easy task. For example, pneumonia used to be called "the old man's friend" because it took elderly infirm people quickly, keeping the suffering limited in terms of time. With that historical background, one can ask if it is appropriate to treat pneumonia in an AD patient.

In my family's case, it would have depended on how far into the progression of AD it had occurred—which would have included consideration as to how that progression had impacted the primary caregiver. For the first several years of his AD, treatment for pneumonia would have been unquestioned. In the last year or so, treatment would likely not have been given.

For the many years in between, this was a hard question to discuss and harder to answer. My family had discussed this on a number of occasions over the years without coming to a definite firm conclusion. Then, my father had a series of small strokes.

His doctors were concerned was that he might have a big one quite soon. Upon hearing this, my immediate reaction was that we should let him go if and when it did happen. However, my mother was absolutely against it. In extremely plain language she insisted that we should do everything to save him, despite the past consensus. When I asked, "But what are we bringing him back to?" She then said, quite simply, what was absolutely true, "I can't let him go like this."

My father did not have a stroke, but there were more discussions about what to do and what not to do. With time and space to think, my mother slowly came to agree that it would be cruel to force him to stay with us through medical intervention in a heart attack or stroke related crisis. I don't know that consensus was ever reached about something like pneumonia or the flu.

Cancer is another condition that frequently arises unrelated to AD but with treatment implications. Again, there are categories within that with potentially different results. If the cancer is of a fast-progressing kind and is terminal, that would influence the consideration one way. On the other hand, many men above the age of sixty-five test positive for prostate cancer. It is usually a slow growing cancer. For an otherwise healthy person, treatment is standard. However, for an Alzheimer's patient, there is a lot of stress involved in simply taking medical tests, having blood work done and so on.

Family Conflict. It is rare that all members of a family view the process and/or progress of AD in their loved one the same way. Old disputes come up. New complaints arise. Judgments are made on each other's conduct as well as on each other's disclosed, hidden or projected intentions.

Family dynamics change dramatically post-diagnosis. Economic issues almost always come to the forefront. Traditional positions of family hierarchy may change. Try to deal with apples as apples and oranges as oranges. Resolve issues first within your own heart and mind. Otherwise, you will be battling with ghosts of memories.

First, allow yourself the space to let whatever arises in your own mind come up without judgment. These are usually conflicting or simply intense emotions. They will eventually settle into some clarity. Let people say whatever comes up in their minds without judging. This is a very important time to keep still. When the dust settles, you can then lead by example and thereby invite family members to also drop their historical grievances.

This is critical because at some point the issue of death and dying is going to arise. If family members haven't worked out their own confusions, then the process of dying for the afflicted family member will occur in the context of chaos rather than support and dignity.

The sooner that issues are addressed, the better. In short, listen to everyone involved in the caregiving circle. It can prevent much ugliness later in the journey. Try to soften everyone's position, especially your own. Don't simply listen to their words, listen to the feelings behind the words. Addressing the feelings behind the words is often more helpful than responding to the words themselves.

Fears of isolation, fears of genetic flaws, simple sadness and depression over watching your loved one disappear in front of your very eyes, are all things that will affect everyone involved, and are often too difficult to express directly. So expect that you, as well as others in your situation, will say or do strange things.

Again, now is the time to forgive past sins and drop old grievances. Use the AD diagnosis as an opportunity to understand that no one has the luxury of waiting. Decide what is truly important right now, and help each other go through the process.

One way to work with conflicts is to simplify the situation by gently asking a direct question: What would each person in the caregiving network want done with them should they be in a similar situation to the patient.

The Alzheimer's Family Manual

This question should not be raised from the point of view of waiting in ambush, of wishing to use their response as a weapon in the conversation about the patient. It should be raised from the point of view of exploring each other's soft spots, each other's fears. Each of these things plays a part in learning to deal with AD in the family.

One of the best ways to create a non-judgmental family atmosphere for the benefit of the AD patient is to express your willingness to honor each other's wishes about potential AD dilemmas. Often the battles within a family are testing grounds for one's own fears. To be able to state unequivocally that you will defend their wishes, whether they are contrary to your view or not, goes a long way.

The Alzheimer's Family Manual

On Medical Intervention

This piece was originally written in response to a devious tactic utilized by some unscrupulous members of the medical community. It was used to manipulate family caregivers in order to receive unchallenged reimbursement from Medicare for tests and treatments that were/are not necessary.

While the vast majority of the medical community responds to the difficulties of Alzheimer's Disease with compassion, assistance, and support, there comes a time for many of our loved ones when continued medical intervention is of no benefit. The question of continuing to intervene without benefit is an issue that needs to be addressed by both family members and medical practitioners in a skillful and compassionate way. It is not simply a position on assisted suicide or withdrawing of life support. It is about how we can allow another human being to experience the process of dying without undue interference.

Compassion suggests that many tests and treatments for unrelated illnesses affecting late stage AD victims be prohibited. From a societal point of view, such funds may be put to far better use helping others in need. My family had direct experience with this issue.

When my father was sixty-eight years old he had suffered from AD for approximately thirteen years, unable to speak for the last several of those. He had forgotten how to chew and was exhibiting many late stage symptoms. He had been cared for at home for eight years and had lived in nursing home facilities for the last five. The last few of those years, he was living in a facility specially designed for AD patients. Far from being abandoned, my mother visited him four to seven times each week. My siblings and I visited him several times each year, despite living in distant parts of the country.

Then-recent news reports were filled with the names of famous people being diagnosed with or dying as a result of prostate cancer. The medical community immediately promoted the testing of all elderly men for this illness. While this is commendable for most of the people at risk, it was ludicrous for individuals such as my father.

In the face of Alzheimer's Disease, prostate cancer or any other unrelated disease is the least of one's problems. More to the point, in my father's case, he became more and more terrified of medical procedures as his illness progressed. Drawing blood for monthly tests would have been traumatic each and every time. Taking medication was also difficult for him. No treatment would do anything to benefit his state of mind, and none of it would create any sense of ease for him.

For patients that tested positive for prostate cancer, unscrupulous health care practitioners would approach the spouse, family caregiver or other responsible person and say something along the lines of: "Your husband/father/brother has prostate cancer and we can help him." This tactic puts caregivers in the position of having to say yes, to treat their loved one at a substantial cost to Medicare, including doctor visits and regular testing to monitor the effects of the treatment, and/or a huge cost to the patient's or his family's financial resources.

This kind of treatment is paid for either by public funds for those with no resources, or will drive those with limited resources to public assistance far sooner than otherwise would occur. The costs continue to mount as the treatment continues, until the patient dies of some other ailment or the cancer becomes uncontrollable.

I am not terribly interested in analyzing the financial impact. If there is no benefit to the patient, the financial question shouldn't even come into play. I have complete confidence that testing and treating a late stage Alzheimer's patient for prostate cancer is simply cruel — to the patient and the family. In my opinion, treating a patient for prostate cancer at any stage of AD would not result in any improvement in his quality of life. In fact, the stress of ongoing testing and treatment would make things worse.

On the family side of the equation, unscrupulous medical providers intentionally place the spouse in the horrific position of having to choose accelerating financial ruin or guilt beyond belief should she decline the treatment. In fact, when my mother expressed her wish that my father not be subjected to even the testing, she was accused of not loving my father, of not caring one iota about his well-being.

Doctors, nurses, and administrators at the facility verbally attacked my mother. They told her that she was an unfeeling, mean-spirited spouse who was willing to just let her husband die of cancer. All of these people knew that she had cared for my father alone in their home for eight years and visited him almost every day in each of the care facilities he had been in.

As neither I nor any of my siblings were present when this happened, we could only speak to those involved after the fact. Their conduct was based on either a corporate policy tied to avarice for the fees they would earn treating prostate cancer or simple, cruel ignorance. Unfortunately, it took the threat of a lawsuit to stop their criticism of my mother.

For our family, if my father were to die of prostate cancer sooner than he would die of AD, that was okay. He had suffered more than enough. If the cause of his death was ultimately to be prostate cancer, so be it. In light of his overall condition, there was no benefit in extending his life by treating any such illness.

I have no idea how many prostate cancer tests were performed on individuals like my father. Given the number of men with AD, it was likely enormous. I was told that every man at my father's nursing home was tested, except for my father.

This is not in any way, shape, or form meant to denigrate the issues facing a man with prostate cancer. If prostate cancer is the only illness facing someone, or if they are likely to regain or maintain a positive quality of life, they should indeed be tested and treated.

But for AD patients, and especially for late stage patients, the question of treating other illnesses needs a reasonable evaluation before engaging in testing and treatment. If my father had broken his leg, immediate treatment would be needed. Setting his leg and administering pain medication in that situation would provide an obvious benefit. But any intervention can and should be evaluated in light of AD, and its progression in a specific patient.

No benefit is to be gained treating late stage AD patients for other terminal illnesses, whether or not they are conventionally treatable. This is a key issue, as on top of the emotional burden, patients' and family finances will only be further crushed by the additional burden of unnecessary treatment.

For society as a whole, the financial issues are of equally great concern. The public money that is being used for people in situations analogous to my father's is wasted. Those funds should be used to truly benefit those in need, whether they are in need as a result of AD or any other illness — or for any other genuinely beneficial purpose.

The Right to Die

This piece was originally written in 1996 when the Right to Die issue was working its way through the United States federal court system. The question has been raised, debated and litigated in other jurisdictions. It continues to be an open issue in most.

In 1996, there were several cases winding their way through the United States Courts of Appeal concerning the so-called "Right to Die." Without going into the separate analyses of these cases or the ones that followed up to the Supreme Court, it was clear that the Ninth Circuit judge who drafted one of those opinions was correct in his statement that this will be as divisive an issue as abortion.

When the Supreme Court agreed to hear appeals of the Right to Die cases, it seemed critical that the National Alzheimer's Association file an Amicus Curiae brief[4], as several other concerned organizations had already stated that they would.

The National Alzheimer's Association declined, however, and after consulting with our local Santa Barbara chapter board, I requested an explanation from the National head office. I received a letter in response from the then-chairman, telling me that because the issue was so divisive at the Board level, the organization could not file

---

[4] Amicus Curiae (literally "friend of the court"). An individual or organization who is not a party to an action, but has a strong interest in the matter, may petition the court for permission to file a brief on the issue. These are commonly filed in appeals concerning matters of broad public interest.

an amicus brief. He stated that the Board believed that for the organization to set out *any* position would put it at risk of self-destruction from the conflicting views within its own membership.

As I wrote to the chairman, I believe it is absolutely necessary to have the discussion on an individual as well as on a family basis. This discussion was then and still remains vitally important to AD families.

I did not then nor do I now feel it necessary to proclaim any particular "truth" about the right to die. There is no good reason to push people in one direction or another. However, I do believe it is necessary for any family circle of support to create a space where the widely conflicting emotions that this issue may produce, individually and in families, can safely be expressed.

There are more than five million people in the United States afflicted with AD. Some are diagnosed in their twenties, some in their eighties and some in every decade in between. Over time, AD progressively devastates their memory, their ability to conceptualize, their motor skills, and their perceptual awareness. There is no cure.

However, people do not become terminally ill with AD. They die when some other illness becomes uncontrollable. The law now permits the holder of a legally drawn health care power of attorney to make decisions about medical treatment for an ill person unable to communicate his wishes. While these powers of attorney sometime extend to treatments for any illness, they are generally prepared to cover terminal illness issues. As noted, AD is not necessarily defined as a "terminal" illness.

My father was diagnosed with AD at the age of fifty-six. He had already been showing symptoms for a few years. For the first eight years after the diagnosis, he was cared for at home by my mother. For the last several years of his life, he lived in AD specialty care units. He was then classified as being in the late stages of the illness.

My father had been unable to speak for several years. On many days, he sat unmoving for hours at a time, but there were periods during which he was so agitated that he was unable to sit still for even a few moments. For the most part, he had forgotten how to chew.

On some occasions, there seemed to be a flicker of recognition. On others, he just sobbed uncontrollably. What is kindness under these circumstances?

To focus properly on the Right to Die issue, it is necessary to understand in a visceral way that once someone is past the early stages of AD, his or her quality of life may generally be described as almost relentless suffering. I invite anyone who questions this to visit AD patients and try to experience their world. It should be a real visit, not a ten minute drop-in, take a peek around and leave kind of visit. Spend eight to ten consecutive hours alone with them.

If possible, spend twenty-four or forty-eight consecutive hours with them.[5]

The patient has no break from AD. They have no possibility of a break. Therefore, you should take no break. Be with them for that extended period without a gap and without any other companion. Do it the next day and then again. With that experience, the true depth of the question, as well as your own answer, becomes apparent.

Many formerly "terminal" illnesses are now treatable. This is true from pneumonia to cancer; from high blood pressure to kidney infections. With many such illnesses, death can be staved off for years. Many illnesses previously deemed fatal can now be completely cured.

In the past, death was often regarded as a blessing, a release from the ravages and suffering of disease. As noted before, pneumonia was called "The Old Man's Friend" because it took you quickly, and somewhat gently, beyond your suffering in this life.

What treatments are appropriate for late stage AD patients with such unrelated illnesses? What is kind? Many diseases we don't consider a problem now are terminal in the absence of modern medical intervention. Should patients be treated for a flu, or should it be allowed to develop into untreated pneumonia?

---

[5] This is unlikely to be permitted at a facility, but can be done at the patient's home. It can be a most welcome break for the primary caregiver while at the same time giving you an unmatched opportunity.

Regardless of the illness, modern medicine can keep an AD patient alive far longer than palliative care, which is pain treatment solely for the comfort of the patient. One must understand that treating an unrelated illness keeps the patient trapped within AD. Is it appropriate to so extend his suffering? This is an evaluation that must be done individually by each family, and each family may come to a different conclusion.

My father was always very clear about his own wishes. I have vivid recollections of conversations that took place in my boyhood and into my teen years. He was explicit that no efforts were to be made to save or prolong his life if he were in an accident or contracted a terminal illness without any real hope of recovery. He wanted no part of such an existence.

He had these same conversations with my mother and sisters. To honor my father's wishes and instructions, I believed it would be appropriate to refrain from treating any illness he might have developed following his late stage AD, to do nothing except to ease his pain. As I saw and experienced him for the last several years of his life, there is no doubt in my mind that to extend his life by any means would have been cruel.

I had no interest or desire in taking affirmative actions to end his life, nor had he ever requested that of me. However, I did think it necessary and was prepared to prevent interference with the natural process by anyone who would intervene to extend his life. The sole exception was my mother. As the primary caregiver for so many years, I needed to support her. The most I was willing to do in terms of intervention was to encourage her to let go.

In any event, so long as my father was willing to eat, I was willing to feed him. If he stopped eating, I was fully prepared to prevent insertion of a feeding tube. Likewise, were he to have become ill aside from AD, I would have prevented treatment other than palliative care. As he was been unable to communicate verbally or even non-verbally for the last years of his life, he was unable to protect himself from modern technology and pharmacology which could extend his life. I carried his instructions in my heart.

As it turned out, my father did not develop any other illness. His body was quite strong and healthy for many years in most ways other than the AD. When he entered the final phase of dying, he had eaten and drunk less and less. The last eleven days of his life, he neither ate nor drank. We gave him small doses of morphine to ease the physical suffering. Eventually, he simply stopped breathing.

Each family affected by AD must come to grips with the final journey based on their own experience and their understanding of their own loved AD patient. Not all people are as explicit in their wishes as was my father. Many may have expressed the opposite desire, which should be similarly respected.

Recalling the prostate cancer issue discussed earlier, I would reiterate that only someone who has seen their beloved AD patient confused and panicked by medical procedures can truly understand how torturous it can be.

And only someone with a loved one suffering from AD, or another such illness, can truly understand that any hoped-for benefit must be seen in the context of the patient's suffering.

If my father were to have died of prostate cancer, of which he showed no external symptoms, it would not have been qualitatively worse than for him than to have died of some other illness. All other illnesses he might experience paled in the face his AD.

In the event that his life could have been extended for six months, or worse, even longer, by treating any non-AD illness, it would have been unkind. In my view, simply because medical technology could maintain his body, merely prolonging his suffering was neither a sufficient nor comforting course of action.

As to the societal and governmental concerns, this view holds for any analysis of my father's health care. Let the money be spent in a way that might genuinely benefit people. It is clear that there are many people whose suffering can be alleviated through the expenditure of health care dollars. My father's suffering in his last years could not.

I do not believe that keeping my father's body functioning through medical intervention until a major organ collapsed beyond our technological skill to repair it would have been kind or beneficial to him. The simple truth is that as a result of having been born, each of us will definitely experience death.

The Alzheimer's Family Manual

Instead of struggling to stave off and delay death at any cost, as individuals and as a society, we can be kinder. For my father, or anyone in his situation, simply by being with him and creating a gentle environment for him, we can assist him in dealing with the process of dying. For, it was dying that he was clearly doing.

I am not suggesting or even recommending that people mimic what I did. I am recommending that people simply support AD patients and their caregivers, and those with other illnesses, in whatever way one can. Visualize their suffering. Try to connect with their experience. Touch it in some way if you can. However you understand it, always be kind.

The issues raised above can logically be extended to the notion of affirmatively acting to end someone's life or not, with the same issues of clarity of intent while a loved one was competent.

No caregiver or family member that I have ever met, spoken to or heard of has ever said anything other than that they would take steps to end their own life, while they were still able to take such an action, rather than go through the AD process. If for no other reason, the issue needs to be contemplated by each of us.

This is an issue raised by many, many children of AD patients who have spoken with me, and an issue with which I personally must remain prepared to face directly. This is and will always remain an intensely personal issue. I would not want anyone interfering with my decision either to go through the entire disease process or to end my life while still competent. Nor would I wish to interfere with anyone else's decisions, whatever they may be. I leave my decision to whatever wisdom I have developed or connected to in my life, just as I leave their decision to them.

This is an extraordinarily brutal issue that demands that we discuss it amongst ourselves and in our support networks. If nothing else, we need to have considered it personally. It is only through that personal assessment, rather than as a philosophical exercise, that one will be able to be kind, and to create an open and non-judgmental space where caregivers, patients, and family members are able to talk about it.

If someone wishes to use every medical technology known to extend their life or whether they wish to end it the moment they are diagnosed, they need a space to express those thoughts in safety, without fear of attack. Having confidence in our own conflicting emotions and the process of working with them, we can allow for someone else to feel the texture of their own emotions. This is a gift that we can only give if we ourselves have felt the textures of our own thoughts and fears.

Children's Issues

In 1992, I attended the annual National Alzheimer's Association conference in Chicago. The last afternoon, all of the participants were invited to the Association's downtown Chicago office. I sat on the bus next to a woman about my own age. She immediately turned to me and asked whether my interest in Alzheimer's Disease was personal or professional. Upon hearing that my father had been afflicted for many years, she told me that her father as well as several of his siblings had it. She then tried to ask, actually demand, to know how I could sleep at night knowing that I might get it too.

As with many children whose parent or parents have Alzheimer's, it seemed that her life decisions at this point were predicated on the fear that she too would become ill. For all children of an AD parent, the weight of the fear appears all-consuming at times. This is a common topic in conversations among Alzheimer's children. It comes out in different forms: whether or not to marry, whether or not to have children, whether or not to move to a new place. Suicide and assisted suicide are common topics.

She was not alone in having sleepless nights. She was certainly not alone in her fear. So I answered her as honestly as I could. I apologized that I had no simple or easy answer for her, for myself or for anyone else. My answer was that I had no alternative other than to rely on my personal spiritual practice and discipline, how I have been trained to work with my own mind.

These issues and fears are heightened when the ill parent or caregiver is having a bad time. For some, it reaches a crescendo at the time of the parent's death. For others, it reaches a crescendo in the period just following that death. Then the issues seem to go underground in one's consciousness for a while. We begin to settle back into the general illusion everyone shares: sickness and death will happen to us, surely, but not right now and not in the foreseeable future. Truly this is an illusion. It gives comfort temporarily, but barely covers the open wound.

****

In a meeting with two dedicated and energetic supporters of Alzheimer's work a year or so later, I suggested that individuals whose parents suffer from AD had different issues than other caregivers. One person had cared for her spouse for many years; another was an Alzheimer's Association local chapter Director. Neither of these individuals had a parent stricken with AD.

My suggestion was instantly dismissed by the spousal caregiver whose concern for all caregivers was truly unquestionable. She told me that I was being ridiculous; they either were or were not going to get sick so they should just deal with it. You have to get on with your life. Essentially, the message was that children should stop whining.

I suggested that she was missing something. This was a woman who spent decades organizing support groups around the world, someone of boundless energy and compassion. I said to her that she didn't get it because it was her husband who had been ill, not her parent. She had no genetic issue in the background.

I told her that I had just been to the oral surgeon for a root canal. She said that she had several and they were awful. I told her that I had been asked if I wanted a gold or porcelain cap. She told me that she had gold because they lasted longer and were overall much better. I pointed out that my first thought, when asked about a gold cap, was the films I had seen as a child in which the concentration camp guards were pulling out and piling up the gold teeth of the Jews.

Her faced turned pale. She was of the age where she would have been one of those Jews if she had been in Europe then. The Director looked at me as if I had made a really fine debating point. I looked at him and said that it wasn't a debating point. I explained that although he understood my point intellectually, but that the spousal caregiver, understood what I was talking about viscerally, in the depths of her body. They both then understood that children of Alzheimer's parents have fears that others do not.

The result was that I was asked to give a talk to a forming support group for children of Alzheimer's patients. As part of announcing the new group, the monthly newsletter of the Santa Barbara Alzheimer's Association, *Side-by-Side* included the following piece I had written:

"In April of 1999, my father's children and grandchildren all went to Florida to say good-bye. He had been diagnosed with Alzheimer's Disease 15 years earlier at the age of 55. Hospice had been caring for him the last few months.

This was an opportunity to say goodbye properly, an opportunity to express love. Most important, it was an opportunity to acknowledge simply and directly our lives together. For my father's grandchildren, in addition to saying good-bye to their grandfather, they were also able to see their parents' loving participation in the process of his dying.

In speaking with my sisters, and with other people whose parent or parents have Alzheimer's Disease, it is clear that, as children of AD patients, we have issues and concerns that differ from other caregiver groups. To put it succinctly, there is not a week that goes by without another news report of genetic tendencies toward, and links to, Alzheimer's Disease.[6]

Under such a barrage, our fears are heightened. Vigilantly watching for our own mistakes becomes ever more preoccupying hyper-vigilance. Jokes by friends, comedy routines on television, and people's offhand

---

[6] The reports usually confirm that a child of an AD patient has a small but increased likelihood of getting AD when compared to someone that is not a child of an AD patient. They do *not* confirm that one will get AD, just that there is a measurably larger likelihood of being diagnosed with AD.

Alzheimer's references when someone misplaces their checkbook, provoke a different reaction in us than for others who do not have the familial connection.

As we take care of our parents and raise our children, we look at our personal calendars quite often. We compare the date of AD onset in our parents with our own age. We do this math while looking at our own children.

Many people have spoken to me of their fears. The first fear that is usually expressed is that they will get sick before finishing caregiving responsibilities for their parents and before raising their own children. Some people have told me that they have had babies in an effort to stave off the fear of their own impending illness by bringing new life into the world. Others have refrained from having children out of fear that they will inevitably become a burden to any such children.

Underlying our fears is the horror that we might have passed on our own potentially bad genes. While in each instance there may be a surface acknowledgment that there is only a tenuous logic to that fear, the underlying panic is not quelled.

There is often an inability to express one's panic over potential AD experiences to spouses, siblings, or friends. A misplaced checkbook or fumbling for a name can trigger a panic attack about early onset for dealing with Alzheimer's in the family. I am quite familiar with that.

The Alzheimer's Family Manual

Whether the response is "Get over yourself," "Don't you think you're projecting just a wee bit much," or alternatively, "Oh, how awful," the gulf often seems too large to communicate across. The difference between people who read news reports about the potential genetic time bombs in their heads and those who simply misplace something in the rush of a busy life is impossible to quantify. It simply exists.

With gentleness, we can be of benefit to those in need, which may include us. Anyone whose parent has AD should explore joining a family support group. Without too fixed an agenda, spending time together can create a mutually safe space to work with one's fears. Know with certainty that everyone in this situation has fears.

It bears repeating that no caregiver or family member that I have ever met, spoken to, or heard of, has ever said anything other than that they would take steps to end their own life while they were still able to make such a decision, if they were diagnosed with Alzheimer's. I have seen personalities both strong and meek insist that they would definitely take such action, rather than go through the process of the disease themselves, or have it inflicted on their family.

Imagining ourselves in the position of our loved ones with AD can provoke profound fear. Taking that fear to heart, we have an opportunity that is truly extraordinary. In our very bones, we can understand that there is no time to waste. Therefore, we can practice forgiveness and kindness beyond keeping score. We can see what is precious in life, and what is unnecessary. In that way, we can honor our parents and the journey that all AD families and caregivers make."

****

The First Meeting of the Adult Children's Group

The first meeting included about twenty-five individuals and couples, all of whom had one or both parents with AD, as well as one professional facilitator. After being introduced as the author of The Alzheimer's Family Manual audiotape, I welcomed everyone and began by noting that as children of AD parents we have different issues than caregivers without any genetic connection. A woman interrupted me after only a few minutes. She announced that she wasn't interested in listening to any of this. She wanted information on how to help her parents, both of whom were ill with AD. I said that I would be happy to give a talk directed more toward general caregiving issues if that was what the participants wanted.

Almost everyone agreed, so I changed the direction of my talk. Within five minutes, one of the participants started talking about how terrified she was that she would get sick before her parents died and would leave a multi-generational problem for her children. She said that she was completely panicked and it was all she could think about. Although she had not been diagnosed, nor experienced any symptoms, she could not bear the thought of her own children being burdened by their grandparent's condition as well as her own upcoming AD. This opened the floodgates. Within moments, the entire discussion shifted back to the original point of the group—issues for AD children.

Some people talked about their thoughts of suicide, their thoughts of having to kill their own parents if they themselves are diagnosed. Some talked about going into the garage and just sobbing. Some spoke of the anger they felt toward siblings who refused to help financially or emotionally, while being quite at ease telling the on-site caregiving child exactly what they were doing wrong.

Even the woman who initially did not want to speak about these things, started to open up.

Everyone in the room spoke very personally about their fears. Would they burden their loved ones as they felt burdened, or would they end their own lives? People were speaking aloud their secret terrors, but not with a view to getting *the* answer, or even just *an* answer. It seemed that the most important point was that the space felt safe enough to voice them at all. No one criticized anyone else's comments or feelings; a rather interesting point given the intensity of emotions surrounding these issues in society at large.

Throughout the evening, people's body language was in accord with their speech, also not necessarily typical. It was wonderful to see spouses/partners sitting quietly, extremely close to each other. Sometimes they were gripping each other's hands but sometimes they were just touching gently. It was also wonderful to see people give each other the gentle space to accommodate the expression of the fears, whether loud or soft, accompanied by no bodily movement to speak of or by sobs shaking their bodies. The atmosphere of dignity and respect was extremely powerful and supportive; again without promising or instructing anything.

Following the end of the meeting, the facilitator asked me privately how I had managed to get everyone to open so quickly and so deeply. She had never seen it happen so fast in any of her facilitated groups. My response was to explain that it had little to do with my interpersonal skills. The reason it happened was that everyone in the room had paid a particular and extremely painful price of admission, except for her. For me, it was my father's illness. While she might have been willing to expose herself in some way to encourage this kind of discussion, it would always be a step removed and therefore not trustworthy in the same way.

Having parents with Alzheimer's Disease, we can be kinder and even more compassionate than those without that connection. Be kind to yourself, to your siblings and your children. When you encounter someone with an AD issue, you have the best tools to be helpful so don't ignore the wisdom you have developed as a caregiver and as a child of an Alzheimer's patient.

Part III
My Father

These recollections of my father concern his life both before and after he became ill. It was written one afternoon in a swirl of emotions when contemplating his life, his death and our connection through it all.

******

Closure seems to be a silly term in the face of death. A body gives one last exhalation and, for the moment, everyone else's struggle of hope and fear ends. Nothing really gets closed except a pair of eyes, and maybe a mouth.

Jerry Weinstein became ill with Alzheimer's Disease when he was about 54 years old. It took him about 15 or 16 years to stop breathing. It might have been longer, but the front he put up convinced everyone around him that things were fine. He hid his illness successfully for quite some time.

Even after he was diagnosed, many of his friends thought that he was really quite okay, that the diagnosis must be mistaken. They told me they had quite clear and wonderful conversations with him, and that he wasn't sick at all.

So, I sat in on a few of their subsequent conversations. My father smiled and nodded at appropriate gaps in the conversation when words, sounds or thoughts eluded him.

The Alzheimer's Family Manual

It played perfectly into his friends' (and all of our) beliefs that their words were worth listening to without interruption. They smiled at me when they left and commented how great the conversation had been. I did ask some of them if they noticed how many words he had said for his side of the "conversation." It was only when they were unsuccessful at recalling anything but the smiles and nods that they seemed less certain about how much of the conversation really involved him.

For my part, I had completely missed enormous hints that something was not right. It started with some strange phone calls. The calls alone weren't so bizarre, it was the reason for them that was weird. My mother would call and start yelling at me, angry that I had stopped calling my father. Apparently, he was very upset that I was no longer calling him.

This was not true: I had been calling him regularly, as I always had. However, saying this made no difference in the conversations. I stupidly thought that it was a simple case of my parents having a hard time adjusting to retirement. I could tell that there was a problem, but, despite my supposed intelligence and education, I couldn't see what was right in front of my eyes.

******

My father had told me that he was bored in retirement. He wanted to work a little bit. It would get him out of the house and also allow him to pick up some extra money. In short, he would feel useful again.

He got a job that seemed perfect. He was hired as a sales clerk at a wholesale electrical supply company. My father only had one item on his resume—that he had successfully run his own wholesale electrical supply business for 30 years. They felt that they had really scored in hiring him.

Unfortunately, he was completely incapable of learning their computerized order entry system. No matter how often it was explained, or what he wrote down, nothing stuck. He couldn't learn even the basics. The word "disastrous" best described the experience for all involved.

Anger and panic seemed to be the bywords in those days. But looking back, so many small things had been ignored that were probably early warning signs. It might be pointless now to think about them because he is dead but, then again, how many of those early warning signs are appearing in me, or in my sisters, or in anyone else I know?

Can I really distinguish with any level of confidence between early warning signs and just run-of-the-mill mistakes? While I cannot be 100% confident, I can still feel the difference between irritation and panic. Panic is a far more visceral experience. It certainly requires an enormous amount of energy to maintain a front to cover panic.

Once again, for me, I am not sure. While walking in the shade of an oak grove on a hot afternoon, I suddenly remember that I can no longer rest in the shade of my father's affection. Opening into that loss extends me in a way that is priceless. I would not cut off those thoughts or cut short such walks for anything. This simple gift of recollection dissolved out from under him.

Ah, my father could smile. He took joy simply in seeing his children or, my goodness, in seeing his grandchildren. And then at a certain point, we noticed that he couldn't quite do it. Before we knew he was sick, his anger and panic seemed to arise completely without reason or context.

He was unable to grasp the street layout near his new home, purchased to enjoy his "golden" years. He started doing things he never had done before, like backing into parking spaces whenever and wherever possible, instead of simply pulling in. He became a spectator rather than a participant in conversations. In retrospect, he was waiting to be exposed and fighting hard to prevent just that.

And then I remember that when I was about 16, he was making lists of things that he had to do. He never used to do that. He always had his checklist in his mind. This was probably about 12 years before we knew he was sick.

Being a typical self-absorbed teenager, I made fun of his having to write things down all the time. I remember that sometime after that, he started carrying around a tape recorder. He told me that he would speak his private thoughts into it while he was driving.

I am haunted by that tape recorder. I can see it so clearly in my mind's eye. I looked for those old tapes everywhere. After he got sick, I listened to every old tape I found in his house, hoping that each was one of those old ones he had saved; hoping for a clue to what his thoughts had been. I never found even one.

I remember going with him to visit his mother in her nursing home. He was still living at home, but he had been diagnosed with AD a few years earlier. When we arrived, he could barely bring himself to look at her. When he did, I thought he would explode on the spot. I never saw such rage and confusion, either alone or together, in a single moment. It was as if an awful joke had been shoved in his face.

He clearly saw that she was older than him and that she was more frail. He clearly saw that she was in possession of her mind, and that he was not. He clearly saw that it was a colossal, horrible wrong.

I loved my father. I was more open with him than almost anyone else. We certainly had our difficulties, periods of not speaking or, just as often, periods of overly dramatic and grandiose fuming. But they always dissolved.

They dissolved because he was braver than me in many ways. He couldn't bear anger between us for very long. Like most teenagers, I could, or at least I pretended that I could. Like most teenagers, I thought I had time and strength on my side. It was far less embarrassing than exposing my faults and admitting my mistakes. He would push such stupidity aside, both his and mine, because it was more painful for him to feel a gulf between us.

His humor was not mean. He took great delight in having us all together to celebrate some event. He got his greatest kicks from setting up a surprise visit by one of his children and keeping it a secret, from my mother or his other children, until just the right moment—when their tension or surprise would be completely ripe.

His anger had the same cascading quality as his love. I am not talking about the anger that appeared when he was hiding his illness, but the paternal anger he had when I was growing up. The engulfing quality made it awful to be on the receiving end. But, it always dissolved. I found it much more straightforward than other, more devious styles of aggression. I think that is why it dissolved so easily. It lacked the gamesmanship so prevalent in many people.

When the thought arose that I wanted to pursue my study of Buddhism in Colorado, I automatically turned to him and told him on the spot. My timing was impeccable as always—we were at a funeral reception. He was furious, accusing me of planning this for a long time, and just springing it on him. I was amazed at how angry he became. I had simply babbled a thought that had entered my mind. I had no particular plan.

When I left six months later to go to Colorado, he arranged a ride for me. His parting words were that it was a cold world out there and he would not send me any money. But, he would send me either a ticket home or to my uncle in California when I stopped this nonsense.

When I was in Colorado, my older sister called to tell me of a disagreement that she had with my father. My sister had just been accepted into the law school of her choice. However, my father had already given a non-refundable deposit to her second choice, the school that had accepted her first. He refused to give up the deposit and allow her to go to her first choice school. On the advice of my Buddhist teacher, I had already made plans to return to college. I would continue my meditation practice while getting my degree.

After my sister told me this, I called my father and told him to give my sister the money for her to go to the school she wanted. I told him that I was sure he had set something aside for my return to school. I assured him I didn't need it as I had saved what I needed for my own college expenses while working in Colorado. He started laughing. He had to admit that he had indeed squirreled away money for my education. I caught him on that one.

When I returned home, I was struck by the depth of concern in his eyes as he looked to make sure I was okay in body and mind. I told him I had been thinking of wearing a skin wig and robes as a joke for seeing him and my mother when I got off the plane. I decided against it as it wouldn't have been funny if either or both had a stroke upon seeing me in that get-up. He laughed, shook his head and agreed that it was definitely funnier as a story of what could have been rather than as an actual event.

He told me that he didn't understand why I wanted to be a Buddhist, but if I did, he was sure I would be the best one. There was such genuine love and confidence behind those words. It still brings warmth to my heart just thinking about it.

During a month-long solitary retreat in 1976, I sent him a letter. I had left my parents' home that summer under difficult circumstances. Having spent about eight weeks pacifying my mother's rage every evening, and experiencing it again the next, I had thought the difficulties were my fault: The aggression was focused at me and my meditation practice. However, it turned out that my parents were having a difficult time in their relationship. I was just a safer, or at least more convenient, target for the household anger.

I wrote the letter in the hopes that I could communicate my basic respect and affection while simultaneously expressing confidence and conviction in my personal path. When I got out of retreat and spoke with him, his open heart and joy at having received the letter was palpable. He had already written back to me expressing his appreciation for my willingness to write such a letter, his appreciation for me as an adult, and finally, the fact that, against my wishes, he had shared portions of the letter with my mother. I think the power of that interchange arose from the open and undeniable connection between us.

Several years later, while I was having dinner with my parents, they were discussing their concerns about my younger sister. They both felt she was having a difficult time personally. I suggested that she could come live with me for a while. My mother was aghast at the idea of sending her into my Buddhist world. But my father said, "Now just wait. I think it has been helpful to him and the idea is worth considering." Such were the different views of my parents.

Their different views came up again when they attended my law school graduation. I offered to arrange a meeting with my Buddhist teacher. My mother's response was that it was a bad idea and that he wouldn't like her. My father's response was again, "Now just wait. I think I would like to meet the person who has had such a strong influence on my son."

When I decided to get married, my mother did not want to attend a Buddhist ceremony. So, my father came to the wedding alone. It was the first time in decades that he had traveled somewhere alone. He came to my wedding because he felt that it was important that he be there for both of us.

He was terribly upset that my mother refused to come. He stayed in a hotel with my brother-in-law, my brother-in-law to be, and my college friend. He hung out with "the guys" in a way he had not since his own youth. He was chaperoned at the wedding by a female friend of my wife whose job was to make him feel at ease.

After the ceremony, when he realized that no one had harangued the attending guests to change their religion, he relaxed. At the reception he met one of my Buddhist teachers, who had performed the ceremony. He immediately put my father at ease by talking about places in New Jersey that they knew in common. This led to people they knew in common.

In response to hearing the name of one of my father's customers, my teacher said, "Hey, I dated his daughter." That ended any issue of his feeling ill at ease. And then, my father danced. He danced, he laughed, and his eyes shone bright.

When I found out that I was to be a father, I called him. I asked if he liked being a grandfather to my nephew. He said of course, he loved it. He was irritated that I would even ask such a thing. I asked if he liked the idea of being a grandparent in general. His response was to ask what the matter was with me. When I informed him of the news, he shrieked into the phone and yelled, "Keep 'em coming!" His joy was glorious to behold.

His AD started a year or two after my daughter's birth. It saddens me that she has no memories of him as a vibrant human being; his energy, smile, and delight. Perhaps this is why I am writing these stories down - before they slip away from me as well. I balance that with my fear that if I write them all down, it would actually seal off his life. Maybe that is the essential mistaken view of closure.

The ramifications of his life impact me continually in deepening ways. To stop that process, or even to think of stopping that process would be to denigrate his memory and his presence in me.

******

I made a special detour to Florida on route to a business meeting when the phone calls from my parents got too weird. I figured that I needed to see what was happening in person. In the garage of their house, my mother told me that he had been diagnosed with AD. Then she fell sobbing into my arms. I needed to be on the spot for both of them so my own emotional chaos had to wait.

When I got off the plane to attend the meeting, I drove in the mental fog that such events produce. When I saw some friends later that evening, they asked what was wrong. I told them what I had just learned and stood there with cascading tears, sobbing more deeply than I ever had before.

The total, absolute loss that was coming was completely overwhelming. I saw hints of the walking corpse to come that would be my father.

******

As he faded over time, being with him became more and more difficult. Still, there were moments; teeing off on a golf course, pointing him in the direction of the hole, the two of us laughing. After five holes, he lined up on the green facing the wrong way.

I called to him and he looked up at me with such sad eyes. I said, "You're tired, let's go home." He nodded in agreement and relaxed because it was clearly okay with me if he was tired. We walked with my arm around him back to the clubhouse and then, hand in hand, to the car.

At one point he was living in a long-term care facility that was beautiful to look at and awful to be in. It was clearly designed for families who liked the idea that their loved one was in a place that appeared to be more of a hotel with nursing attendants than a nursing home. Despite the ice cream parlor (open every afternoon at 4!), the pretty couches and artificial flowers from the interior designer's hotel palette, it wasn't any hotel you would want to stay in.

When I went up to his room, he looked at me as if I were a piece of furniture. He was walking, clearly very agitated, so I started along with him. Up and down the halls. They could only have been a few hundred feet long but we walked them for hours, approximately six of the eight hours I was there that day.

He would go at almost a running pace about halfway down the hall, then stop, gasping for air, huffing and puffing. He was clearly seeing something that I could not, under attack by something that I couldn't help to subdue. He dragged me by my arm for hours, up and down the halls.

About an hour into this, he stopped for a moment. He was breathing hard in the midst of his intense struggle. And then he saw me out of the corner of his eye and BINGO. He recognized me. He smiled at me and then looked at me quizzically, as if to ask how I had gotten here. Then, off he went again.

At dinnertime, they strapped him into a geriatric chair, tying his hands to the chair. He pushed the chair backwards into the wall with his feet and kept pushing, over and over. The staff person showed me where he had broken the wall doing that same repetitive pushing a few weeks earlier.

The staff insisted that he had to be tied into the chair. I couldn't stand it and took him out of the chair. I preferred to continue cruising the hall exhausted than watch him struggle against the restraints.

When it was time for bed, four large female orderlies came in to get him ready. They turned the lights low. Two spoke to each other in Spanish, two spoke to each other in Creole. I have no idea what they were saying, but none of it had to do with my father. As they started to pull his clothes off, while laughing and cackling to each other, he began to push them away with his hands and kick at them with his feet.

The largest and most senior orderly glared at me. She pointed out to me what a bad uncooperative patient he was. I told her she would kick, too, if she were in a dark room with four large people she didn't know, speaking languages she didn't understand, and pulling her clothes off. I had them leave. I calmed him down. He was quiet and in nightclothes within ten minutes.

I had come to the facility because I was told he was being "restrained" in his bed at night, that he was being tied up "for his own protection." I left that evening more exhausted physically and emotionally that I ever remembered. But all I could think of was that while I was able to take a break, he couldn't. There were no eight-hour shifts that ended a day for him. Never had it been so clear that there is no escape from your own mind.

We usually perceive the world in mostly the same way that others do. But my father was trapped in a way that was impenetrable. Whatever he saw, I couldn't even glimpse. Whatever he heard, it passed right by me. Whatever he thought, it grabbed his mind and wouldn't let anything else in.

He was in the most expensive facility we knew of and could afford in the area. He had gone there because it was supposed to be the best. We found another place and moved him as quickly as possible after my visit.

******

Two days before my father exhaled for the last time, tension was enormous for everyone. For the previous nine days, the family had been told by the hospice workers that he would pass away within two hours, or maybe last up to twenty-four. A few days of hearing that same message every morning and evening would make anyone a bit edgy.

I encouraged my mother to avoid going to see him as a death vigil. I suggested she tell him that she loved him, tell him that it was okay for him to leave, and then go home. She refused. Once she got to his room, it was impossible to get her out.

While there, the pain and anguish she felt was everywhere. It was undeniable on her face, in her speech and all over her body. She would watch him breathe, her own body gasping with his. There was the look of complete impotence on her face. In truth, there was nothing she could do for him. Yet she could not leave, despite the stress and very real danger to her own health.

Late that afternoon, as she left the room completely distraught, I followed her out with the idea that I might try to comfort and be there for her. Maybe just hold her hand. She turned and grabbed me with her hands and eyes. She instructed me to go in and put a pillow over his head because, "No one should suffer like this."

From my point of view, for the first time in so many years, the grasp Alzheimer's Disease had on him had slipped away. He was no different than any other person in the last days before death. It was not that he was in so much pain, she was. The simple inhalation, albeit odd enough rhythmically, was all he did at that point. She took it on as her struggle.

His suffering had peaked and plateaued over the course of the last ten or so years. But now, as his mind was separating from his body, so was the grasp of the illness. He seemed quite calm outside of the physical struggle to breathe. His calm, for once, was a clear counterpoint to the state of mind of his visitors.

I told her as kindly as I could that I would not do that. I said that he was not suffering at this point beyond the normal experience that everyone goes through at the end of life, and that the pain she was feeling was her own. She asked me if that was true, or if I was just making something up to calm her down.

I encouraged her to just sit with him and breathe in and out. If she did that, she would see for herself. She tried and seemed comforted a bit.

******

My father used to disparage his own intelligence and other good qualities, as if they didn't really count for all that much. Loyalty, genuine affection, and compassion all seemed pretty good to me. Many of the people I knew who were supposedly intelligent, rich or had some other so-called desirable qualities appeared, for the most part, to lack those very things.

My father seemed to be always saving kids from drowning either at a beach or at a pool. Nobody else I know ever did it with that kind of regularity. My sisters and I would be sitting by a pool gabbing and idly looking around. We would hear my father coming with his transistor radio on. And the next sound would be the radio hitting the concrete, and then a splash in the water as he dove in to pull out some child who had fallen in.

Curiously, the parents almost never thanked him. It was as if that would be an admission that they had been neglectful. But it never bothered him, it was just the way things went. Even after he was diagnosed with AD, he was the one who spotted his grandson in trouble swimming in the ocean. Though he could no longer race in and pull him out, it was his warning that likely avoided a tragedy.

And he could dance, always able to lead his partners just at the edge of their ability to follow. He looked so happy spinning and moving. He could make any klutz look good on the dance floor.

Dancing with his daughters, he was the embodiment of delight. Dancing with my mother, his movements were so assured and so elegant. For her part, she never looked so soft and comfortable as when dancing in his arms.

******

When my younger sister got married, my father still lived at home. I offered to take care of my father for the four days I would be in Florida for the wedding. It was my gift to my mother, she would be "off-duty" for twenty-four hours each of those days. For me, it was just a brief taste of my mother's experience of the past several years.

I was awakened several times each night as he got up, turned on the light, and started to take his pajama bottoms off. Then, stopping halfway down, he would pull them up almost all the way. Then, he would start to take them off. This happened over and over again. Blearily, I would ask him to pull up his pajamas and go back to sleep. I would tell him it was still nighttime. He needed that guidance.

The Alzheimer's Family Manual

There was a funny, comfortable feeling when he would lay in his bed in the late afternoon. The TV would be on in another room. He would go into the same pose he always took watching TV so many years ago, when I was a kid. His hands clasped over his stomach, head supported by the pillow, legs straight out. He was looking straight at the TV in his room while listening to the sound of the TV in the den. It all looked so normal except for the fact that his TV was turned off. It made no difference. I almost felt like I could protect him for a short while—he felt safe for those moments.

At the wedding itself, he did okay until about halfway through the reception. By then, he was confused and exhausted. He asked me to help him leave. As we walked to the car, he stopped. He became angry at himself, and then unsure as to whether or not anger was appropriate. He felt that he should not be leaving. He knew it was a mistake but he didn't know quite why or what he should do about it.

I told him that there was no mistake. It was fine to leave. It was too much energy for him to handle. He clearly wasn't up to being in that environment anymore with music, noise, and people he no longer recognized. It was his last public appearance.

******

At times, I am able to rest in his memory. I find it interesting that I am ready, willing, and able to spend time with the parents of my friends. Often, I am more willing than they are. I am comfortable listening to an old man's stories that he has repeated hundreds of times to his own children, but which are fresh and new to me.

But it is more than that. It is knowing that my father got sick before he reached that point. I am afraid there were so many old stories he never got to tell me, even once or twice. Maybe, for me, hearing someone else's father tell stories is like someone craving alcohol when there is only juice in the refrigerator. It's not quite what you're hoping for, but it is the closest thing around.

The Alzheimer's Family Manual

Part IV
Contemplating Alzheimer's

Being with an Alzheimer's patient over time, one can watch a mind misfire occasionally, then more often, then almost continuously. As the journey progresses, one sees that mind degenerate to the point where it only occasionally, and then barely, connects to simple sense perceptions. In this age of scientific progress in medicine, a body can be maintained for an excruciatingly long time with or without a mind. This is a terrifying thought for anyone who has watched a loved one's mind disintegrate under the assault of the disease.

Caregivers who reflect deeply on the nature of AD and its impact on the patient, the family and the extended network of caregivers, tend to have softer hearts and consequently more empathy for everyone involved. While it might seem odd to think of meditating on a mind collapsing in upon itself, the following contemplations are exercises in deep reflection that I have done in the past and continue to work with.

If these exercises are indeed done as contemplations, rather than simply being read and considered in a surface manner, they are far more helpful. Try to spend a minute or two — or perhaps even just a few slow breaths — and sink into the state of mind as described, step by step. In approaching them this way, the contemplations enable you to get a sense of the experience of being trapped by this illness in a body. They will give you a feel for that experience of one's mind misfiring, with the sense gates opening to the wrong pathway.

With these experiences in mind, you can generate even more compassion when your loved one follows you too closely for hours at a time, giving you no space. With these experiences in mind, you can generate kind thoughts when you are asked the same question every three minutes, no matter how often you have answered.

The purpose of these contemplations is not to generate a resolution of any kind, nor to give you an answer. Rather, it is to put in focus the kinds of thoughts which arise as the result of having a spouse or life partner whose parent suffered from AD. Allow your emotions to arise as you progress through the contemplations. Feel what might be very conflicting emotions.

I am not suggesting that you force any of these contemplations. It is more like allowing the contemplation to deepen on its own despite one's best efforts to keep the feeling at a safe distance. Start with a simple contemplation: the particular suffering of forgetting a word. Because everyone does that now and again, it is an easy place to start.

Contemplation on Words

For this contemplation, imagine that forgetting a word is not an occasional experience. Imagine that it happens all the time...

Imagine the interruption of the internal dialogue we all keep if words aren't accessible any longer to support it...

Then imagine trying to speak to someone else when you can't find the words. Instead, there is just a big gap...

Imagine them staring at you with an expression that is half grin and half irritation with a growing subtext of concern in their eyes. There is tension in the air as you fight for a word, any word, to fill in the gap...

There is tension in the air as they wait for a word, any word, to show that you simply spaced out the word you are looking for...

Imagine that the hole in your mind is nakedly exposed. Think about how much safer it would be to not speak other than to say yes or no. Think about how much easier it would be to just fill in the pauses left by another's random comments because "yes," "no," and "hmmm" can get you through a lot...

Then imagine that the words spoken to you stop making sense. The sounds themselves cannot be distinguished as having meaning...

Finally, while imagining the look of fear and sadness on the faces of the speakers, imagine that the sounds of speech are indistinguishable from any other noise in the environment: It is all just sound...

After letting go into the experience of indecipherable noise, gradually pick out intelligible sounds and come back your normal experience of words. Carry with you the recollection of disconnection. This recollection will enable you to extend out to an AD patient who is losing their auditory reference points. Remembering this experience will enable you to understand more deeply how safe an AD patient feels when you guide them with soft sounds and a gentle touch.

The point of this contemplation is to start to connect with some sense of the specific suffering that AD entails. In actual fact, it is true for all of the sense organs and perceptions — not just sounds.

****Contemplation on Writings****

Consider the written word. The letters are fundamental. We use them to define ourselves when we write our names, to locate ourselves when we go from one place to another, to connect to our world through newspapers, notes, email and iPhones. If the lines we draw, which make up the letters, cease to have coherent meaning, what then? How do we mark our names? How do we note our birthday, our telephone number, or where we live?

This disconnect with the written word can be approached in two ways. You can comprehend the individual letters without understanding the meaning of the words they form, such as reading a foreign language phonetically when it is written in a familiar alphabet. But you can also try to imagine that the letters of your name appear to be written in a foreign script. For example, "compassion" is easily understood by someone familiar with English while Сострадание, التعاطف or 同情 might seem unintelligible – even though they each mean the same thing.

****

Imagine that the letters of your name, which are so familiar and grounding, appear to be written in a foreign script, like the Russian, Arabic or Chinese in the previous sentence....

Imagine looking at your driver's license. Let your mind relax: when you imagine the face on the license, allow it to remain unfamiliar...

As you look at the letters on the license, each time you automatically organize the shapes into a recognizable word, allow yourself to let go further so that you only see the shapes—the squiggles, curves and lines that have no inherent meaning anymore...

Who are you now?

After a while, allow yourself to organize the shapes into normal perceivable forms of letters in your native language.

The Alzheimer's Family Manual

Contemplation on Thoughts

With regard to thoughts, consider the following contemplation:

Recall the experience of being lost in a thought...

Now recall the experience of coming back to the present moment...

Notice how coming back to the present moment is dependent upon a firm recollection of who and where you are. Now imagine that there is no firm recollection to come back to...

Whatever arises in your mind, for whatever reason, is all you have...

Whatever fearful thought arises, there is no recollection of a firm "you" in a firm place to come back to...

There is no way to comfort yourself...

Try to place yourself in that realm without checking in on your recollection of you, on your recollection that this is merely a contemplation...

Now imagine that you are trapped in a dream...

Like a dream, every thought is an entire universe with random activities, hopes and fears. The recollection of a firm "you" is the awakening from the dream. Imagine that there is no firm you to reassure yourself that you are awake...

Instead, imagine being trapped in whatever dream or nightmare unfolds...

The only thing you have is the present thought. Despite grabbing onto that present thought, it dissolves out from under you just like in a dream...

So you try to grab yet another one...

Over and over this happens but nothing really holds...

We are usually the ones on the outside, seeing the effect of the Alzheimer's. We are like the one who is not dreaming, desperately trying to awaken the sleeper. It is no stretch of the imagination to know that we cannot awaken them: We can only enter their dream as best we can and touch them.

With this in mind, open your heart further. When your own fear arises, imagine how much more frightening it is for someone who can't come back. Then open further.

****Contemplation on Being a Child of an AD Parent****

I was walking on the beach with a friend of mine, a doctor with whom I had been discussing Alzheimer's Disease. His father-in-law had recently been diagnosed and was soon to be moved from home to a facility. We spoke, I made some suggestions based on my experience, and then he said with genuinely compassionate curiosity, "How does it feel to walk around knowing that you might have a time bomb ticking in your brain?"

****

To glimpse the fear of an Alzheimer's child, imagine your parent showing Alzheimer's symptoms at a specific, particular age. Pick a relatively young age, perhaps the age of 54, a not uncommon age for this to happen. In fact, that is about when my father became ill. Recollect your own age and count how many years it will be until you will be 54...

Think of the things undone in your life; the obligations to your own family which will still remain after that age...

Imagine your fear of abandonment, knowing the consuming and long term quality of the illness in terms of money, energy and grief...

While your mind may be strong in the present moment, recall that as the illness progresses, your strength of mind will become shaken and start to collapse...

Know that decisions you might make with your present strength of mind are dependent on your confidence in who you are. As the fear that your confidence will dissolve begins to arise, allow the waves of panic for the past, panic in the present and panic of the future to wash over you...

Experience that for a while...

****

There is no time to waste, no time to leave important tasks for some imaginary later. In particular, there is no time to hold onto grievances. Most people feel embarrassed to apologize. They are convinced of either the rightness of their cause or the bad faith of the other person. This completely misses the point that wrong and right sides of grudges don't matter in the face of losing one's mind. It is the negativity of connections to others that needs to be assuaged. Who may be right and who may be wrong is meaningless if there is no resolution of the heart.

If the fruition of this contemplation is to realize that there is no time to carry a grudge, there will be benefit.

Contemplation on One's Own Children

One woman I met refused to have children despite the wishes of her husband. She felt that her father's Alzheimer's diagnosis proved that she likely had "bad genes." While it was possible that the bad genes would show up, this was an awful but bearable thought because she could always choose to exit her body, assisted or otherwise. However, if the bad genes were to show up in her children and they developed AD, that would be unendurable for her.

Those outside the caregiving community are often surprised to know that there are people with AD being cared for by their own parents. In light of that, this fear is not as groundless as one might think. While it is a small risk, it is indeed a risk.

Another woman I know had a child later in life in large part because she felt that it would force her to ward off Alzheimer's. The idea was that the drive to protect, nourish and nurture a child would push her to keep the disease at bay. She grudgingly admitted that such logic was tenuous at best, however, the compulsion was not based on logic and was overwhelmingly powerful.

A third woman I know proclaimed that she was going to tell her children that they were not to look after her if and when she was diagnosed with Alzheimer's. She had told her husband that she was not going to put her family, meaning him and their two children, through what she was going through with her AD stricken mother.

Exactly how and when she was going to tell her children was vague. It was an uncomfortable topic despite the prior proclamation. It was equally uncomfortable when the issue was raised as to whether or not her husband or children would accede to her request should she fall ill. After all, she might no longer have the capacity to argue that or any other point.

With these things in mind, there are two contemplations one might explore. The first has to do with your own child becoming ill:

Imagine that your child, as healthy and happy as anyone else's child, has long since launched his own life....

The Alzheimer's Family Manual

They might have a family, a career, hopes and dreams. Your desire for their happiness, and the desire to protect them from suffering is as intense as it was when they were first born...

But time has passed and it is likely that they will soon be taking care of you...

Then, imagine that they are changing in unpleasant ways...

They become angry for no reason, they seem to be losing things and even getting lost in familiar locales...

They are becoming distant in the middle of conversations...

Then imagine that they are diagnosed with Alzheimer's and all their difficulties fall into their logical, if extremely awful, place...

Now imagine that you, in your old age, once again have to take care of your child...

Your finances, your energy, your whole world is once again consumed with taking care of this child. Only now, there is no hope for the future, there is only fear of what will befall that child when you pass away...

****

Experience that for a while and then emerge with

appreciation of the depth of love you have for your children.

The second contemplation to explore has to do with you becoming ill.

****

In this contemplation begin by imagining that you are beginning to see the same signs in yourself that you saw in your Alzheimer's parent. Perhaps you begin to stumble on even ground. Perhaps you panic when you misplace your checkbook and are then embarrassed later when your checkbook is right in front of you on the table, even if no one is home to see...

Perhaps you forget which road you took home; or maybe you forget which road will take you home...

Imagine that you start writing notes to yourself as reminders, and then as more than reminders...

Let the fear arise that you are starting the Alzheimer's progression...

Imagine that you are frightened to tell your spouse, or anyone else, for fear that either they will dismiss you as a hypochondriac or for fear that they won't...

Now imagine seeing your children...

Would you have the strength to ask for their help in

living if that is your wish?

Would you have the strength to ask for their help in dying if that is your wish?

Imagine the fear of knowing that you will forget their names, their faces, their joys and sorrows...

Imagine the fear that you have bequeathed this same illness to them...

******

Contemplate for a while and, again, recognize the depth of love you have for your children and the desire to protect them from pain.

Contemplation on One's Spouse

Being married, traditionally and in most people's view, is intended to be a life-long commitment through sickness and in health. Given that this illness is unlike a short terminal disease, one needs to consider whether or not you would wish to put someone you love into a position of having to care for your body, with you trapped inside it somewhere.

Before making any snap decision, spend twelve, twenty-four or even more consecutive hours with an Alzheimer's patient, if possible in a care facility. This is not to criticize any specific facility, or even to critique institutionalization as a method of caregiving, because many are quite good. For many people individually and for society, there is no other option. The purpose of such an exercise is to try to touch the world that an Alzheimer's patient lives in—the one that they cannot escape. In all likelihood there will be a range of cognitive capacities in the facility. Just experience it for a while, but definitely not just ten minutes or even just for an hour.

Spouses have it pretty rough. One of the difficult twists of the times in which we live, is that there are profit oriented economic forces at work in the hospital and long term care industries, some of which are discussed elsewhere in this book.

Personal economics also come into play—as any long term care situation can bankrupt a family, for some people there is a distinct economic advantage to divorcing an Alzheimer's spouse. This indeed was suggested to my mother. While there may be logic to the economic aspect of such a suggestion, the personal issues of abandoning one's sick spouse, even if it is merely a matter of form and not substance, can bring emotional devastation.

Being married to the child of an Alzheimer's patient is not an easy situation. You can't allow your spouse too much indulgence in panic but on the other hand, you can't eliminate fears. The fears cannot be eliminated because 1) they are not based on conventional logic so logical arguments will be unsuccessful and often counterproductive; and 2) it might not be hypochondria.

While watching the decline of an ill in-law, a spouse

should be strong and supportive. After all, for the spouse it isn't very different from any other illness. The problem is that the potential genetic component isn't in your gene pool. Therefore, you might take the attitude that everyone just has to live their life and "we" will deal with whatever happens when it happens.

Instead, consider the contemplations previously described to get a feel for the kind of mind-set that can arise in your spouse. Then, do the following contemplation:

Imagine that your spouse is forgetting things a bit...

They are getting testy when asked about events of the day...

Imagine sitting home waiting for your spouse to return from the grocery store because it has been a little too long; then perhaps an hour or two too long...

Imagine rushing to the door when you hear the car return, thankful that there has been no accident. But nothing is said, there is no explanation. No story of long lines at the store, or going to do an extra errand or two, or of meeting a friend and having coffee. Only a frozen space...

Imagine that this is not the first time...

Knowing that his or her parent had Alzheimer's, do you say anything?

Can you say anything which won't be heard by your

spouse as the most horrible, threatening accusation imaginable?

How long do you wait to raise the question, if you raise it at all?

How many times do they have to lose the checkbook or their car keys, or lose their way home to force you to raise the question?

Then imagine what it will be like to have to take care of your spouse, perhaps for decades...

Perhaps your spouse has always said they wished to be cared for at home until they pass away...

Contemplate the changes in the nature of your own life...

Then imagine that your spouse wishes to be abandoned by you in an institution to live out their days without them "inconveniencing" the rest of your life...

Finally, imagine that your spouse wishes to commit suicide, and desires your help...

****

Recognize that the depth of your emotional responses, conflicting or otherwise, expresses the depth of your connection to your spouse.

Without understanding that these scenarios run

through the minds of every Alzheimer's child at some point or another, it is not possible to be a genuine source of support. Without understanding that these are real issues for an Alzheimer's child's spouse, there is no way to talk about them when everyone is capable of cognizing the potential choices and results.

Once again, I am sorry to say, there is no safe harbor other than kindness. It is empathy, not trying to force an agreed upon result. It is based on allowing the warmth of your shared space to be a gentle anchor that can accommodate the mental turmoil that such thoughts generate.

Contemplation on Siblings

Each child in our family has their own logic as to why they will be the one to get Alzheimer's. My older sister expressed her view that it would be her, because she is the oldest. My younger sister felt that it would be her because she looks most like my father's side of the family. As for me, I am the only male...

None of these logics has any genuine basis of certainty yet all of them haunt us in their own way. It is the amorphous quality of the way one is attacked by Alzheimer's that generates that haunting. For a long time, any of us could have the same forgetfulness that "normal" people have. But the question always remains as to whether our forgetfulness is of the normal variety or not.

With that in mind, imagine that you are very close to

your brother or sister...

Indeed, they are the only one(s) who truly share your memories of your parent, of who your parent was before they manifested AD. Imagine the grief you share in a way no one else can share with you...

Then knowing that each of you is somewhat more at risk than the average person for getting Alzheimer's, imagine that one of you will get it...

Imagine the effect on that one and the reactions of the others...

Then switch places so that you have imagined each one of you with AD...

Then consider, if one of you had to get it, who would you would want it to be...

Then, as one face flashes in your mind, feel the guilt if it is not you. Feel that groundlessness if it is...

Without punishing yourself either way, generate compassion towards yourself and your siblings...

Rest in that.

The Alzheimer's Family Manual

Contemplation on Working with Panic

When fear and panic arise in oneself, it is easy to see how you search out a reference point to confirm or undermine the panic. Imagine fear and panic arising because you lose your reference points. There is nothing available to undermine the panic.

When fear and panic arises in someone else, it is easy to see how your response affects them. If you panic along with them, it confirms that their panic is justified. If you don't go along with the panic, however, it serves as a stabilizing influence for them.

Knowing that the progression of AD serves to undermine strongly held beliefs, decisions about what to do cannot be delayed. There is no precise moment qualifying as "This is it." Any delay will heighten the risk of your ability to make decisions being taken away from you.

With that in mind, contemplate the effects of remaining alive with this illness...

Contemplate the impact of terminating your life...

Contemplate the effect of absolutely no medical intervention; not for flus, colds, strokes or any other illness that is life threatening in this time of scientific progress or otherwise...

In other words, contemplate all of the issues that may arise in the Alzheimer's journey...

*** Facing One's Fears ***

It is difficult to be brave enough to expose one's own fears. Being brave enough to be nakedly exposed is hard in the best of times. But, any other approach will definitely leave decisions in the hands of others. That may be okay for some and anathema to others. Sometimes it is easier to be brave if there is no other genuine option. In any event, it is best to see where your support circle of family and friends are, and it is best to see that now.

It would be cowardly for me to end this section without stating my own thoughts and wishes. This is not to urge anyone in one direction or another. As I have previously said, it is necessary and kind to support whatever decision another person within your caring circle might make—whether one is in agreement with it or not. That being said, while there are people who wish to stay alive as long as medically possible, for religious or secular reasons, perhaps in hopes of a cure which will bring them back their life or simply out of fear of death, I am not one of them.

I have asked those who I love and trust, and who love me, to assist me to continue my personal spiritual practice for so long as I am able. Then, no different from any other being, I would seek to avoid the suffering that I cannot manage. I hope to exit from this body gently in a warm supportive environment. It is my hope and prayer that I will know when to start my last journey. Knowing that there is no safe harbor, perhaps I will, perhaps not.

Afterword

Whatever work I have done in the Alzheimer's world since the onset of my father's illness, is my attempt to repay and pass on in some small way the many kindnesses I have been shown by my own family, friends and fellow travelers. I hope it will be of benefit to Alzheimer patients, parents, children, and caregivers—both family and professional.

It was through the guidance and extraordinary efforts of my teachers on the path, the Vidyadhara, Chögyam Trungpa Rinpoche, his Vajra Regent Osel Tendzin, the Venerable Khenchen Thrangu Rinpoche and the Dzogchen Ponlop Rinpoche that kindness was awakened in me. Their wisdom, clarity and insight was instrumental in helping me work with my father's Alzheimer's journey and helping me support other patients and caregivers as they traveled similar roads. I dedicate whatever merit generated by this work to the benefit of all beings.

The Alzheimer's Family Manual

Resources

The most important direct resource for patients and caregivers is the local chapter of the Alzheimer's Association in the United States, and other affiliated Alzheimer's organizations in Canada, the UK, Europe and throughout the world.

Equally important is the Alzheimer's Association itself. The website is www.alz.org/. On that site, you can search and find contact information for your local chapter.

There are many helpful books for Caregivers. In particular, *The 36-Hour Day: A Family Guide to Caring for People Who Have Alzheimer Disease, Related Dementias, and Memory Loss*, is an incredible resource, with one proviso: This is a book that should be used as an encyclopedia rather than something to be read like a novel. There is great information in it that can be overwhelming to someone who has just learned of the diagnosis of their loved one.

Other Caregivers — wherever they may be found — are invaluable companions on this path.

The Alzheimer's Family Manual

The Alzheimer's Family Manual

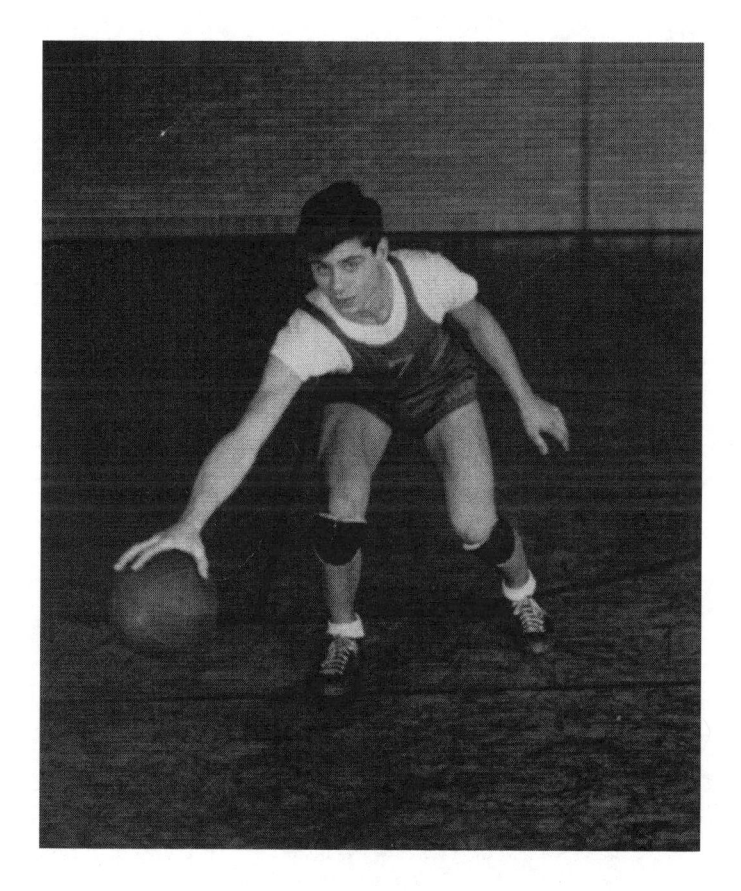

Jerry Weinstein
1927-1999

Made in the USA
Middletown, DE
16 June 2015